THE
MEDITATION
SUTRAS

How To Create and Maintain
A Daily Meditation Practice

RUCHA TADWALKAR

ISBN: 978-1-7358793-0-7 (paperback)
ISBN: 978-1-7358793-1-4 (e-book)

Edited by Cathy Suter
Book cover and interior design by Jasmine Hromjak

First edition published 2021.

Published by Shanti Path
www.theshantipath.com

DEDICATION

I invoke the blessings of God, my guru, and my parents. I humbly bow down to your unconditional love. I will never be able to repay you for the blessings you have showered me in this lifetime. I dedicate this book to you.

My immense gratitude to the support of my friends who I consider to be family. I would not have had the strength and perseverance to write this book without your encouragement. I am lucky to have you all in my life.

BLESSINGS

May everyone's paths be guided by the light of auspicious virtues and noble deeds. May you understand your life as an opportunity to release yourself from the bondage of mental suffering. May everyone realize the divine bliss that already exists within.

Om Tat Sat

TABLE OF CONTENTS

CHAPTER 2

Preparing the Mind 65

CHAPTER 4

Changes and Realizations Evolving
from a Daily Meditation Practice 181

PREFACE

I started meditating when I was ten years old. My father taught me *Japa Mala* Meditation, a technique used to concentrate the mind by utilizing the beads of a necklace to repeat a *mantra* (sacred syllables or words). He showed me the proper way to hold the *mala* (necklace) and explained how to use the beads to chant. He helped me to pronounce the mantra correctly and shared its significance. It was actually my dad's own meditation practice that helped to guide mine. He told me to sit every day in front of our home altar and that this practice would help me throughout my life.

I began meditating every night. But, like many people, my practice became inconsistent over time. If I missed a day, I told myself I would do it tomorrow. There were phases when I would meditate every day for a few weeks, before again my practice faded away. Sometimes, months or even years passed before I meditated again.

As I grew older, I began to observe that on the days I did not meditate, emotional reactions and conditioned thinking easily overcame me. I felt imbalanced and quickly agitated. My mind would be everywhere else but in the present moment. I realized that, unlike any other activity, meditation always helped me feel centered and peaceful in my life. So, I made a commitment to myself to not only continue meditating, but to stick with a daily practice

At the time of writing this book I have not a missed a day of meditation for over six years. It is due to this consistency that I have been able to handle unexpected circumstances with calmness and remove certain emotions like jealousy from my mind. It is by doing the internal work every day that I have been able to notice the oneness in all and transcend many selfish desires. It is because of meditating each day that I have become more creative, insightful, and self-aware. It is through the gradual reconditioning of my mind that I have learned to not take things personally and discover my true nature as not this individual ego. It is because of my daily practice that I was able to recognize my guru as a genuine spiritual guide and receive his blessings through *diksha* (initiation) on this path. Through my experience, I can confidently say that turning the mind inward every day is the key to inner happiness.

In *The Meditation Sutras* I share the exact methods I have discovered, learned, and adopted in keeping a daily meditation practice. Anyone who regularly implements these techniques will not only be able to sustain an everyday meditation habit, but also move toward uncovering lasting inner peace.

INTRODUCTION

What is a *sutra*?

A sutra is a thread of knowledge that can be elaborated on. In ancient India, the *guru-shishya* (teacher-student) relationship was based on this traditional method of teaching in the *gurukuls* (schools). Since spiritual and religious knowledge was transmitted to students orally, a sutra made it easier for a disciple to not only commit to memory what was taught, but also for it to become deeply entrenched in the mind. For this reason, a sutra could be defined as a simple sentence that can easily be recalled. The intention being that if the sutra (statement) can be remembered, then the knowledge expanding on it would also be thought of immediately.

The Meditation Sutras is not *only* meant as a guide, but also to help affirm and reinforce what you are already realizing through your own daily meditation practice. It is strongly advised that you not just merely open the book up, read its contents, and satisfyingly tell yourself that you have now learned how to create and maintain a daily meditation practice. Rather, the knowledge in this book should go from being abstract to instinctual through your direct realization of it.

If at any time you read something that does not make sense to you, come across some new concept, or have any doubt about what has been written, then I encourage you to continue with your meditations. Find out for yourself whether you can answer your own questions, satisfy your curiosities, and remove uncertainties.

Initially, not everything written here will be easy to comprehend. We can only make sense of something from our own level of understanding. And, there is no greater place where that stands true than when it comes to religion and spirituality. It requires personal experience and an intimate understanding.

Similar to how the experience of enlightenment can never be wholly conveyed with words and descriptions because it needs to be experienced, the process of meditation can only be fully understood through practice. I can tell you about the benefits of meditation and how it will transform your life until my face turns blue and I run out of air. But, will that bring you any closer to experiencing it for yourself? Will that help you to understand the different ways in which meditation can create an internal change? You have to willingly participate and realize it for yourself.

Daily meditation steadily guides us in examining every aspect of our lives with honesty and clarity. Silence is necessary in order for us to gain insight and perspective into ourselves. We must have self-awareness before we can begin to create any inner changes. Conscious living requires constant internal inquiry and solitude.

The Meditation Sutras provides a detailed system on how a person needs to utilize and direct their energy, time, and efforts in order to maintain a daily meditation practice. Through the consistent application of these comprehensive methods, one will not only sustain a meditation practice, but also steadily get closer to reaching inner happiness.

What has been written in this book comes from my direct experience of Vedanta. The Vedas are known to be the oldest religious texts in the world. In Sanskrit, *Veda* means knowledge, *anta* means end. Vedanta signifies both the end of the Vedas, as well as that portion of knowledge that contains the universal principles and practical methods to uncovering one's blissful nature, known specifically as the Upanishads. Due to their timeless wisdom and application, Vedanta has come to form the basis of *Sanatana Dharma*, eternal way of living or eternal principles. Today, this path to self-realization is known as the Hindu religion.

If you read any of the books forming the core of the Vedanta school of philosophy, composed of the Bhagavad

Gita, Upanishads, and Brahma Sutras, you will find the same foundational knowledge within those texts as in *The Meditation Sutras*. What makes this book unique is my direct realization of these philosophies and practices. Although *The Meditation Sutras* is an original book in that I have created the framework and system to develop a daily meditation practice in the context of modern life, the basis of this knowledge comes directly from Vedanta. For this reason, whatever you read here is not abstract and intellectual knowledge or my opinions and theories. I have merely made the time and effort to go within and discover the truths of these sacred books for myself. Anyone can do the same.

You will see the phrase "Key Vedic Concepts" after each sutra. This means that the sutra contains certain principles from Vedanta. Since almost nothing written in this book is new information, almost everything can be traced back to the roots of Vedantic knowledge. For those interested in learning more about the source of these practices, a Vedic dictionary has been provided in the back of the book.

Importance should not be placed on the number of the sutra, rather more attention should be given to the sutra itself and the content that expands on it. The structure and format of the book have been laid out so as to make it easier to understand the material. The numbers of the sutras are intended to guide a reader and help one to logically make sense of the content.

The Meditation Sutras has been designed to slowly take a person from the obvious to the subtle. In other words, from external attention to internal awareness. In this way, each chapter builds on the last.

Ideally, this book should be read in the same sequence as it has been written. Chapter 1 sets the foundation for a meditation practice by clarifying misconceptions and providing direction. Chapter 2 gives a detailed explanation on how to cultivate the mind for meditation. One needs to first know, understand, and start to implement this knowledge before they can proceed to develop a practice (Chapter 3) and realize the benefits (Chapter 4).

The pace at which you read this book will be determined by the consistency of your practice. The level at which you have synthesized this knowledge with your own personal experience will guide you in how to allocate your time in reading each sutra. It could be that while you are already practicing and realizing the benefits of certain sutras and do not need to spend much time reading them, at the same time you are attempting to intellectually understand others. In addition, you may need to read some sutras several times or go back to previously read ones so as to understand them in a different way. This completely aligns with the writing style of the book.

You will find words, phrases, and concepts repeated in various sutras throughout *The Meditation Sutras*. This has been done on purpose. In order to make any point clear, it bears repeating. Explaining methods and practices in different contexts helps give a textured understanding of the material. For this reason, a lot of the information overlaps and connects with the other chapters.

Whether you are new to meditation or an experienced practitioner, *The Meditation Sutras* has the ability to speak to those at all levels of their practice. In this way, the book is a valuable resource in helping you progress from wherever you are in your journey.

It should be noted that *The Meditation Sutras* describes only *some* of the changes that may be experienced as a result of a daily meditation practice. This book gives general descriptions of how a person who continues to meditate with dedication and faith may naturally evolve. Although inner changes will happen, how they will look and when they will occur differ with every individual.

CHAPTER 1

Purpose of Meditation, Foundational Understanding, and Clarifying Misconceptions

1.1 NOW, TO CREATE A DAILY MEDITATION PRACTICE.

This may be your first introduction to meditation. As a beginner, it is important to gain as much knowledge as possible as you step onto this path. Being informed to the best of one's abilities is always commendable when starting any journey. Preparation will help you avoid misconceptions and overcome challenges, as well as begin with clear understanding.

Conversely, you may be a seasoned meditator. However, until this point you may have tried to create a daily meditation practice, but found it challenging to keep it going. You probably started very enthusiastically and with good intentions. Most likely you began to sit regularly, but due to time, obligations, laziness, discouragement, or lack of proper guidance, you stopped your practice along the way.

Perhaps you are reading this book because you found meditation to be helpful in getting you through a challenging period in your life. Possibly you discovered it as a means to help you recover from a specific type of trauma or as a tool to help you relieve stress. Many people discover meditation during times of upheaval in their lives or as a novel concept with which they can experiment.

Unfortunately, many do not maintain their meditation practice after feeling like they have overcome their hardship. Once feelings of anxiety dissipate and some normality begins to be experienced again, meditation becomes less prioritized, maybe even done away with completely.

Soon though, discomfort appears again. Perhaps, this time an obstacle shows up in a different way. A new setback happens, or something from the past replays in the mind. Maybe a set of expectations go unrealized.

Sense enjoyments and material objects are sought after in hopes of giving one that endless happiness. When they go unachieved or the initial satisfaction of attaining them fades away, then disappointment, sadness, and frustration take over again. Once more a strong desire for mental relief arrives.

No matter how an individual discovers meditation and why they begin a practice, one common thread weaves through most people's experiences: they are unable to keep a consistent meditation practice going over time. This happens even when an individual very much wants to meditate every day, but still cannot somehow sustain a practice.

The average person returns to meditation to help them feel more peaceful, then does away with it when they feel a remote sense of calmness. As a result, one goes from feeling satisfied one moment to feeling disappointed the next. Riding these emotional waves comes to be seen as a normal part of life. It does not occur to most people that there is a way of permanently removing this cycle of pain and pleasure through daily meditation.

The mind acts as a filter for each experience we have and depending on the quality of our thoughts, either creates a positive or negative impression. Why is it that two people can have the same experience, but be affected differently? Our relationship with the world depends on how we already keep our mind.

An everyday meditation practice has the potential for fundamentally changing the pattern of our thoughts. By bringing awareness within, we begin to observe our internal dialogue. Through this process, we come to understand what our mind chooses to focus on and the kinds of thoughts we entertain.

Why do certain thoughts keep recurring? Why is a particular situation bothering me? How is my past affecting my attitude today? How is what I am thinking and feeling preventing me from moving toward real happiness? What kinds of limitations am I placing on myself because of how I view my life? Through this level of self-analysis we begin removing the barriers to our progress.

The mind has to be slowly guided to sit without distraction. As we withdraw the senses from external focus, we reduce the number of thoughts. We re-train the mind to not be led away by every impression that enters it. We become selective of the kinds of thoughts we encourage and reinforce.

An everyday practice has the potential to eliminate negative thinking and emotions altogether. Can you imagine never feeling greed, jealousy, or anger because they have stopped arising within you and not because you are suppressing them? Joy is lived, not as a conscious decision, rather because it has become a person's character.

Daily meditation transforms a person from the inside out. To rewire the brain requires inner work that cannot be completed in a short amount of time. Since the depths of our minds are limitless, undoing life patterns requires traversing the sprawling terrain of our past impressions. This is not a simple task that can be achieved in a quick manner.

Neither is it a pleasant experience to unearth the sources of our suffering and inner conflict. This is an ongoing process that requires one to openly face their limitations. Many stages of growth have to be endured before one can arrive at a place of sustained equanimity. Each individual needs to undergo the necessary levels of their own self-development. Only with consistency can a person transcend these blockages. It is for this reason that meditation has to be a daily practice. One has to continuously work on lifting the mind higher and keeping it there.

An inconsistent meditation practice does not allow one the time to gradually create internal changes. Instead, meditation becomes a tool to temporarily relieve oneself of uncomfortable feelings that eventually come back again in one form or another. To create permanent change a person needs to get to the root of their thoughts and emotions.

Creating a regular practice should not be confused with meditating for longer periods of time, such as once a week in place of every day. It is better to slowly cultivate an ongoing practice, than to have one extended meditation session every once in a while.

Consistency means every day, without interruption of practice. The intention is to slowly work on keeping the mind concentrated for longer periods of time, not to see for how long one can meditate. Over time, meditating becomes not only easier, but also joyful. Naturally, one feels like increasing the duration of their meditations.

Meditation should become a daily habit like brushing our teeth, bathing, or eating. These are all a given in day-to-day life. Meditation should become such a regular part of one's daily routine that a person does not sit and think about whether they should meditate or not. In order for meditation to become second nature, we have to intentionally work on it every day.

Daily meditation is a way of gradually coming back home, greeting the soul after a long time, recognizing a familiar feeling of peace that only silence can bring. We create an everyday practice to recondition the mind, end the cycle of joy and sorrow, transform our thoughts, realize oneness with universal Truth, and merge with infinite peace. These are not things that anyone can teach or demonstrate, they have to be directly experienced through a consistent meditation practice.

KEY VEDIC CONCEPTS: *Abhyasa, Prayatna, Sadhana, Sthiti*

————Footnote
Now: Patanjali's Sutras, Brahma Sutras, each chapter of the Bhagavad Gita, and many other scriptures in Sanskrit begin with the word, *atha*, meaning, now-then. This is completely intentional and for a purpose. Atha, connotes that we are mentally prepared to begin at this moment. This both reaffirms our commitment and prepares us for the journey ahead.

1.2 THE GOAL OF MEDITATION IS SELF-REALIZATION.

There is one constant that never changes due to time and space. It has no beginning and no end. It has always existed and will continue to exist. It has no boundaries or limitations. It is infinite, everlasting, and omnipresent. It resides within each and every person, waiting to be discovered.

When the mind is free of all thoughts in the height of meditation, everything becomes one and there are no boundaries. Our true nature of love reveals itself when we are aligned with the supreme consciousness, which we always want to come home to, but are too caught up in the outer involvements of this material world to recognize.

When one realizes the divine presence within and acknowledges that same higher nature in all, differences disappear. Personalities and characteristics are understood in their true light as different impressions of the mind. When all identities fall away, only oneness exists.

What is there to take personally or feel jealous over when we understand that this body is a temporary vehicle perfectly selected for each one of us to learn our own karmic lessons? When we realize that each experience is an opportunity in helping us reach that ultimate freedom, anger and greed lose significance.

A self-realized person treats everyone and everything as part and parcel of oneself. Where there is an internal understanding that individuality and form are only misperceptions of the mind, separateness ceases to exist. Where there is no other, there can be no fear of another. Fear and freedom can never go together. Until this oneness is realized, there can be no peace among humanity.

We can only see oneness in all by first realizing it in the self. This does not happen through the eyes, rather in the heart. True knowledge of the self takes one beyond narrow understanding through the senses. For the majority of people, whatever can be taken in through the ears, eyes, nose, mouth, and skin is accepted as Reality. However, only a person with direct experience of our real unbounded and limitless nature knows Truth to transcend the restrictions of body and mind. It is the experience of oneness that penetrates the spirit and helps a person to know inner peace.

Inner peace does not waiver with circumstance. It is not determined by what is happening to you or outside of you. Peace is a permanent state of mind. It is who we are in every moment. It is the way we already keep our mind. This natural state becomes revealed to us through our own self-efforts in meditation.

Being peaceful should be a result of one feeling peaceful, not out of obligation or compulsion. It should develop from one not knowing any other way of being in this world other than with fullness of heart. Compassion follows from having done the inner work to reach that level of understanding within oneself.

Self-realization can be known as many things, such as enlightenment, moksha, liberation, or nirvana. It can also be called equanimity, inner peace, permanent happiness, inner freedom or our real nature. No matter the word or term, the concept remains the same, the realization that we are not this individual consciousness, but that one universal Truth.

Higher understanding will gradually dawn even in someone who is not inclined or interested in reaching the goal of self-realization. Although the initial motivation to practice meditation may be to get some mental relief and alleviate stress, a daily practice will change a person. It cannot be that an individual who meditates every day will remain the same. The personality, attitude, and habits will undergo a shift and be reshaped. It is this self-evolution that takes one from being a person of suffering to realizing expanded consciousness.

The goal of meditation should never be to show others how much you have progressed or how enlightened you have become as a result of your practice. Neither should one misunderstand their gradual self-development and growth to mean they have overcome human suffering. There should not be a mere suppression of hate, anger, and worry. These feelings do not just go away. Eventually, they come to the surface because they were never exhausted. Such a person does not live in freedom. They are still bound by the shackles of the mind.

Although a person may feel temporary relaxation and stress relief through daily meditation, the goal of meditation should always be to live (consistently) in this world with equanimity. One should be driven to meditate by a desire to realize ultimate peace. Merged in silence, the mind becomes quiet. A person of inner stillness maintains evenness of mind no matter their relationship with external circumstances. Someone absorbed in a state of tranquility naturally lives in a higher frequency even while participating and engaging in the world.

Meditation is unlike any other experience a human being can have in this life. It cannot be understood through the senses. We cannot imagine it because it goes beyond the realm of what we know through the body, mind, and intellect. Neither, can it be described with any reference to past experiences or wholly encapsulated with words. One has to directly come to know it through their own practice. As much as one can speak of the sweet taste of sugar or the beautiful sight of a sunrise, one must actually experience these things to fully appreciate them—it's the same with meditation. The mind becomes illuminated with the wisdom of self-knowledge.

This is one of the most important sutras in the book because it establishes the goal of meditation. One must understand the purpose and intention of meditation in order to be able to maintain an everyday practice. It is important to know what one is continuously moving toward. This sutra serves as the roadmap and vision on the journey to realizing our true nature. If the goal of meditation is self-realization, then what ongoing adjustments do you have to make within yourself to reach that ultimate Truth?

KEY VEDIC CONCEPTS: *Anadi-Ananta, Brahman, Moksha, Roopa, Svadharma, Yoga*

1.3 ALL HUMAN BEINGS HAVE THE RIGHT TO SELF-REALIZATION.

Human beings have the privilege to be able to meditate. Elements, plants, and animals do not have the ability to choose what they think or how they live. Instead, they are guided by their natural instincts. The nature of fire is to be hot, the nature of a tree is to provide shade, and the nature of a lion is to hunt. None of these have the capacity to be something different. Fire cannot decide that it wants to be cold and have the ability to freeze.

However, human beings are equipped with a higher consciousness than the animal mind. We have the capacity for rational thought and discrimination. We have the ability to cultivate understanding, shape our perspectives, and determine the type of attitudes we keep. We have a choice in our quality of life and the values we practice. We make deliberate decisions each day to either respond thoughtfully or react instinctively.

Ancient teachings tell us that the human body should be kept healthy in order to have the energy to direct to spiritual pursuits, such as meditation. Unfortunately, when most people have energy, it gets spent in daily responsibilities and obligations, as well as engaging in sensual pleasures and recreational activities. Granted some activities are necessary to our essential well-being. However, even maintaining bad habits such as smoking, gambling, taking drugs, and other addictions use up our limited physical energy.

When one has the vitality, it should be directed to exploring the mind and attempting to elevate the consciousness. We must learn to use the body and mind for the purpose for which it has been given to us by making time for inward study. By intelligently using our cognitive and physical abilities to raise the self, we move closer to experiencing our supreme nature. The more diligently we apply ourselves toward this goal, the faster we progress. Every person has been granted this opportunity, whether they choose to use it or not.

Although one may have limited capacity to discriminate due to mental disabilities or unrealized potential in this life, through their own karma they can naturally evolve into elevated states of consciousness. One must continue applying themselves in whatever way possible during this lifetime to end the cycle of suffering and begin the path to liberation.

We must not waste this human birth. Anyone willing to put in the time and effort can realize inner peace. Meditation means unceasingly trying, every day, to work toward realizing our higher nature. As long as one never gives up the thought of the divine presence within, all of one's actions will be directed toward realizing the ultimate goal of supreme Truth.

KEY VEDIC CONCEPTS: *Abhyasa, Karma, Prayatna*

1.4 CONFIRM YOUR EXPERIENCES AS YOU MEDITATE.

Any knowledge we have of the higher realms of the mind comes from the direct experiences of those who have explored their own inner consciousness. Yogis before us, who have sat in consistent and disciplined introspection, have discovered that by directing their physical energy inward, the oscillating mind can be completely transcended.

Through their realizations we know that the cycle of pain and pleasure that all humans inevitably experience in this lifetime can be eliminated. We do not have to wait for an afterlife to put an end to our suffering. Sustained happiness, the kind that can never be taken away, can be experienced while we are still living in this world within this very human body. The requirement is our willingness to go within and work toward it through our own efforts. With a steady meditation practice, we can ultimately uncover the purpose of human existence and realize our oneness with a higher consciousness.

Until you begin this journey yourself, this book will make very little sense to you. You will only be able to fully realize what is written here insofar as your direct experience of it. Otherwise, it will be abstract, intellectual knowledge that only sits in your mind for a few seconds, but does nothing to change your inner nature.

Telling yourself you do not have time, ability, or knowledge to meditate are only ways of trying to convince yourself to not do it. A first-year medical student cannot possibly perform surgery. However, with specialized training, education, and practice, this individual gains the skills to one day perform an operation. It is still the same person. Over time with persistent hard work, they acquired mastery over a new understanding and gained a different perspective. They had to start from somewhere.

Similarly, with meditation, you have to begin from where you are now. To properly grasp the content contained within these pages, you must have your own daily meditation practice. Only through consistent practice, will you naturally come to understand and appreciate what has been written here.

You should be reading, studying, intellectualizing, experimenting, implementing, and analyzing yourself continually, alongside meditating every day. Reflecting on what you have read, thinking about if and how it applies to you, and making attempts to integrate these philosophies helps knowledge to become your own through the direct realization of it.

The words contained in this book should give you the framework and language in which to make sense of your practice, as well as the changes you are seeing as a result of meditation.

This book will help you stay on course when you begin to doubt your practice and your faith weakens. These pages will further encourage you to keep going on your journey toward self-unfoldment.

Abstract knowledge can only become lived experience through application and integration. When higher knowledge has fully penetrated into one's very being, a person no longer has to consciously think about what is the correct way to live because spirituality has become a part of their character. It is this direct experience that instills an unshakeable faith. Being able to verify what you have read through your own personal experience of it is like proving a theory correct.

Without this gradual and organic self-discovery, any changes you experience will be temporary. Reading about someone else's spiritual journey may help motivate your own practice. It may also provide comfort in humanizing your own experience and what you are already feeling. However, merely reading and thinking about meditation will not serve you. It can only affect you to a certain extent, beyond which your own inner work is required.

Pure study, without practice, cannot lead to internal transformation.

Without direct understanding, the most well-intentioned aspirants become vulnerable to misdirection. Those without lived experience grow fanatical, expound dogmas and doctrines, follow others blindly, hate people who follow other religious and spiritual paths, and engage in endless arguments. The only way to put a stop to these quarrels is by experiencing Truth in oneself.

In fact, dedicated meditators may not have to pick up one spiritual book in their entire lives because their own meditation practice guides them and helps them realize the right path to the self. But, to come to the same realizations within as what has been written in sacred texts mandates a very strong disciplined and consistent (read: daily) meditation practice. This is the only way to reach the goal.

Self-discipline should not be viewed with antagonism or disgust. Disciplines for the body tend to be seen as negative and limiting. However, it is mandatory for spiritual advancement.

Just as there need to be rules and regulations on the road to prevent accidents, and electricity has to be channeled properly in order to be effective, one cannot gain control over thoughts without bringing the body and senses under restraint.

Changing what you think and how you think has to be done by you. You alone live inside of your head. You are the only one who knows what goes on there. You can fool others, but you can never escape your own mind. So, this work cannot be outsourced. It has to be taken up by you alone.

This book is meant to be practiced. You do not need anything outside of yourself to take up meditation and do it every single day. The only way to fully realize what is written here is to have the lived experience of it. If your intention is to read it, try to only make sense of it intellectually, or use it as a resource for your academic study, then please put the book down now and go about your everyday life as you have been.

KEY VEDIC CONCEPTS: *Jivanmukti, Sadhaka*

1.5 PRACTICE THE SAME MEDITATION TECHNIQUE.

Moving from one type of meditation method to another does not give a person an opportunity to develop focus and delve deeper into the consciousness. When the meditation method keeps changing, obstacles arise. Energy and time are taken up in getting used to a new practice, learning the method, wondering if it is being properly practiced, doubting the technique, wondering if it is really helping or a previous method should be tried, or a completely different one altogether. All of this defeats the purpose of attempting to make the mind quiet and concentrated.

The same meditation technique must be practiced every day. It should not vary from day-to-day, week-to-week, or month-to-month. A person will have to experiment to find the best method suited for their temperament, personality, and natural disposition. Whatever meditation technique is ultimately chosen, it should be one that resonates, feels the least challenging, and can be easily applied to oneself.

What one concentrates on during meditation will vary from person to person. The focal point chosen should invoke in one a feeling of lightness and complete absorption. Whether it is the sun, a deity, or the breath, cultivating unconditional love and devotion to the chosen ideal helps to raise the level of the mind and improve quality of thoughts. Meditating on a noble sentiment such as happiness or the well-being for all of society, instead of our personal joy, can also bring us to a higher vibration. The quality of the object, words, or symbol one chooses will start to become a part of the individual personality. Whatever ideal one holds in the mind, a person will come to imbibe those attributes and begin to inherit those same qualities. Therefore, although there are many choices in what one can use as a point of concentration, it is important to remember that the method chosen will over time penetrate the consciousness.

Initial struggle will exist, no matter how carefully and intentionally a meditation technique has been chosen. The mind may wander, perhaps there may be some physical discomfort. When one is not used to bringing awareness within and developing one sole focus, challenges will inevitably arise. It is a natural step toward elevating the mind.

Many people get bored with their chosen meditation technique. They tire because there is no excitement or change. This indicates that the mind is still gravitating toward external sense pleasures and attraction for variety. In this stage, the mind can easily get drawn back into conditioned patterns. So, every effort must be made to maintain a disciplined and rigorous practice.

One should do their level best to create a *sadhana*, the same daily spiritual practice. Real yogis meditate at the same time of day and practice the same meditation method, while gradually building on the duration, day in and day out. They are incredibly devoted to their practice. Finding a technique that is best suited to an individual's unique character and disposition makes maintaining the same meditation routine less difficult.

KEY VEDIC CONCEPTS: *Nitya, Sadhana*

1.6 IF YOU DO NOT UNDERSTAND YOUR CHOSEN MEDITATION TECHNIQUE, DO NOT PRACTICE IT.

The meditation technique one chooses to practice should make reasonable sense to the person utilizing it. It should be well thought out and understood. One should make efforts to learn how this particular method helps to focus the mind. Whether concentrating on the breath, focusing on a symbol, repeating a mantra, or any other technique, an individual should know how to correctly practice it and why it leads to deeper states of quietude.

Many people begin practicing meditation because of a friend or family member. They hear about the benefits someone has experienced and decide to try that same type of meditation themselves. They figure that if this technique has helped this person, then it should also create the same effects within themselves.

We often look to those who are already meditating, imitating their practices without fully understanding why a person has chosen a specific method. Sometimes a person may have experimented with numerous ways of meditating to find the one suited to their temperament.

Other times, one may have been initiated by a master or guru and given a particular meditation technique because it was deemed appropriate for their disposition.

Although enthusiasm is absolutely necessary in sustaining a daily practice, that same execution may or may not be efficient or productive. We all have different personalities and natural inclinations that draw us to different styles of meditation. Some types are less difficult for us to adopt than others due to our innate character.

If one is blindly practicing a meditation technique without foundational understanding, it can have adverse effects. It can leave one feeling discouraged and empty, as though a promise for peace went unfulfilled. It can cause disappointment. When one feels that a particular method does not result in anticipated benefits, the frustration from it can cause one to stop meditating altogether.

These expectations should be managed by properly understanding the meditation technique. Learning how this particular style of meditation will benefit a person and how to practice it correctly will not only make it less challenging, but also improve the chances of being able to maintain a practice over time.

KEY VEDIC CONCEPTS: *Shraddha*

1.7 IF YOUR CHOSEN MEDITATION TECHNIQUE CAUSES CHRONIC PAIN AND DISCOMFORT, DO NOT PRACTICE IT.

Experiencing chronic headaches, dizziness, and nausea are not natural outcomes of a meditation practice. Neither are having insomnia, anxiety, or tension after meditating. Persistent sickness or constant nervousness could be signs that someone is sitting for meditation longer than the mind and body are ready for and that more preparation is needed. It could also mean a person is forcing themselves to practice a style of meditation that does not resonate with their personality. Additionally, it could mean one does not have the proper guidance. It may also point to other serious physical and mental health issues that need to be handled with medical care and sensitivity.

A person should immediately stop practicing their chosen meditation technique if they experience ongoing adverse effects from their practice. One can try other meditation methods. However, if after trying a couple of different meditation styles this does not eliminate the issue(s), one should stop meditating altogether until the source of the problem has been found.

Meditation should make a person feel calmer and more relaxed. Steadily, the mind feels lighter and elevated. Granted, some minor physical challenges may be felt due to not being in practice of sitting for long periods of time or in certain postures. These are initial adjustments that many people face when beginning a meditation practice. However, meditation should never cause ongoing discomfort or pain. If an individual experiences enduring ailments, this could indicate a deeper issue.

One should choose a meditation technique that they find comfortable and relatively easy to grasp. There are various ways of concentrating the mind. Any practice one chooses should be suited to their character and disposition. There are many paths available that take into consideration the multitude of different types of personalities in human beings. It is critical that one thoroughly understand and wisely choose a meditation technique. Correct practice of meditation should gradually help a person feel peaceful and develop a balanced mind.

KEY VEDIC CONCEPTS: *Prayatna, Shanti*

1.8 CLEAR QUESTIONS AND DOUBTS.

One needs to ask as many questions as needed about meditation and the method they have chosen before applying it, and even while practicing it.

Ignorance grows when one does not seek answers to questions. One should feel completely satisfied by the information received, otherwise doubts and frustrations will impede a meditation practice.

Additionally, holding onto assumptions about the benefits of a particular meditation technique, such as how it will change an individual, can deter a long-term practice. Having expectations of certain results only produces more confusion in the mind and makes one weary of meditation in general.

One should do their best to seek out trustworthy teachers and resources, as well as learn the correct intention and application of their chosen meditation technique.

A person has to be absolutely clear on what they are doing, why they are doing it, and how one should properly approach their practice, otherwise it will fall apart easily and quickly, and could cause harm.

KEY VEDIC CONCEPTS: *Ajnyana, Avarana*

1.9 MEDITATION IS A CONSCIOUS PROCESS THAT REQUIRES PATIENCE AND PERSISTENCE.

This world is not designed for a daily meditation practice. It offers too much excitement. There is always some new activity to try, a different place to travel, or a novel adventure to be experienced. Even in daily life we crave exotic pleasures in food and drink. We are always fascinated by what more we can engage our senses in and the variety of ways we can do it.

With the world being so inviting with all of its objects and material desires, it will not support one in creating and maintaining a daily meditation practice. If we add the ongoing challenges most of us face with work, health, and relationships, this material world is the last place to encourage and nurture quiet solitude. This only means that one has to cultivate such a strong determination for their meditation practice that nothing will deviate them from pursuing their own divine nature.

Just as if one were learning to play an instrument or speak a new language, meditation takes ongoing effort. Gradual movement forward requires patience and persistence. Meditation necessitates active participation. One has to regularly practice bringing attention inward.

When someone is sleeping, the mind is not available to them; it is completely shut off from the world. Unlike sleep, where the mind is not aware of itself, in meditation the mind is not absent. One is aware of the condition of the mind, whether it is troubled and excited or calm and quiet.

In meditation, one is purposefully engaging with the mind to lessen thoughts and make it quiet. Using drugs in meditation does not enhance a practice, rather only takes one farther away from understanding the real nature of the self. One cannot have command over the mind when the mind itself is not present.

Intoxicants will not help one to permanently overcome anger, greed, and jealousy, rather they obstruct the process to realizing true inner peace. Substances cannot rid a person of attachments and desires, which must be transcended on the path to inner freedom. Pills and stimulants do not help cultivate evenness of mind, a natural outcome of a regular meditation practice that helps us to live in this world with equanimity. One cannot apply a temporary solution to create a permanent change.

Meditation should never be approached as an escape from confronting emotions. It must clearly be understood that no shortcut to inner peace exists. One has to consciously go within to move from being a suffering individual to being free from the restrictions of the mind. We come out of our misery through self-efforts. A passive or indifferent attitude does nothing to help us raise ourselves to a higher level. It is both unfortunate and a mistake when someone limits themselves through external, temporary, and sometimes dangerous methods to realize happiness. We have the potential and power inside of us to reach an exalted state of bliss that any external method cannot produce.

With a consistent meditation practice, lower-base thinking and conditioned patterns start to fall away. The subconscious becomes replaced with the faculty of reasoning and conscious decision-making. By developing mental keenness, slowly the temptation to occupy the mind in senseless outside engagements subsides. Naturally, the intellect becomes strengthened through a daily practice. Having such restraint over the mind is necessary to guide it from restlessness to stillness.

This happens in steps during meditation. At first, the mind will wander. Over time, one develops focus. Naturally, the mind will move back and forth between drifting and concentrating. Gradually, one will be able to hold the mind at one point. Again, it will move from a stream of focus to being distracted. One will experience different states of consciousness. These stages are necessary to prepare the mind to reach the final abode of oneness. This takes time and perseverance. We gradually build and organically realize the results of a meditation practice through constant application.

The higher consciousness always exists in us whether we are occupied in our daily lives or not actively engaged in any action. We just are not aware of it because we have busied our minds with external things. For instance, whether a blackboard is filled with words or not, the blackboard still exists. Similarly, whether the individual consciousness is filled with thoughts or not, the supreme consciousness always exists inside of us. In meditation, purifying the mind of emotions and thoughts is like wiping a blackboard clean. It enables us to recognize the divine nature within that has always existed. For this process to take place, the mind has to be alert.

In meditation, we are moving toward becoming aware of awareness. With a daily practice, we gradually start to become conscious of ourselves in all of our activities. As we perform our tasks with alertness, we become a witness to our actions and thoughts. This helps us to see our imperfections and flaws. Through this awareness, we realize what needs to be changed within ourselves. We modify our behavior. We raise our own standards. We cannot help but be more productive, conscientious, and efficient. As a result, we move through life with serenity and balance.

KEY VEDIC CONCEPTS: *Buddhi, Dharana, Dhyana, Prashanta, Sakshi*

1.10 GOES BEYOND RELAXATION.

One must feel relaxed in order to meditate. A tense body does not allow a person to become aware of the natural flow of breathing or take in deeper breaths. Releasing tension in the muscles helps to circulate the blood flow. Letting go of tightness in the body helps to withdraw the senses from the external and bring awareness inward.

This is why Vedic philosophy includes such practices as *Abhyanga*, *Yoga Nidra*, and *Shavasana*, among many other relaxation techniques, as preliminary options on the path to meditation.

In our modern day, we use the phrase "self-care" to refer to the time we make for relaxation activities. Self-care gives us time to unwind and give ourselves a break from the other stressful parts of our lives. Most self-care practices involve engaging the senses in the outside world. Relaxation has become synonymous with using objects to derive pleasure and experience interim relief. This provides a respite from the responsibilities of life.

Without undermining the importance of taking care of oneself through enjoyable activities, rest, and hobbies, as long as we rely on anything external to give us temporary satisfaction, we continue falling into the same pitfalls and circumstances that keep us in the cycle of needing to take a break from our everyday lives.

Many people view meditation as a form of self-care. While there is nothing wrong with this, this perspective inherently limits the purpose and intention of a meditation practice. Meditation has become popularly known as a way to help one feel relaxed and calmer because very few people get past this stage. The potential to transform the inner spirit and rise above the agitations of the mind far surpass these surface-level benefits.

The question must then be asked: why delay looking at the root of our tensions when we can remove the very source of our restlessness?

Meditation is similar to physical exercise. When you exercise, you do not see weight loss immediately, it occurs over time. You may feel better, have more energy, and a desire to eat healthier, but the transformation happens after following a regimented routine. Similarly, with meditation one feels more relaxed by giving the mind a conscious respite, but the deeper changes evolve over time.

A daily meditation practice takes us beyond relaxation. It permanently restructures the brain. When we fundamentally change our thought patterns, the way we live also changes. Meditation creates space in the mind to consciously think about how one is interacting with and relating to the world. When the mind has too many thoughts, it cannot begin to think about self-improvement and change. When the mind is quiet, one can discriminately think about one's own behavior. There is clarity in thinking.

Daily meditation enables a person to get rid of sorrow, instead of putting internal challenges on hold to deal with at a later time. An everyday practice helps an individual to move from acting out of habit and reaction to living with awareness. Removing conditioned thinking and unhealthy patterns frees the mind to accept the present moment. Automatically, one begins making healthier decisions because one's mindset has shifted. A person naturally becomes self-reflective, gains a positive perspective, and takes actions toward realizing the higher self.

As daily meditation reconditions the mind, the need to separately create a space in one's life to alleviate stress becomes unnecessary. Each thought you allow in your mind, every decision you make, the way you treat yourself and others, all become a continuation of your meditation practice. Daily meditation removes the need for intentional self-care because one's entire life becomes a spiritual practice. When a person is living each day with purpose and intention, what is there to take a break from?

KEY VEDIC CONCEPTS: *Abhyanga, Shanti, Shavasana, Yoganidra*

1.11 NOT AN INTELLECTUAL PURSUIT.

Any new information learned must first be understood on an intellectual level. A person needs to logically and reasonably make sense of any knowledge in order for there to be an appreciation of it. This applies in meditation as well. Thinking about theories and various meditation practices, understanding the philosophies and purposes behind meditation, learning how to correctly implement techniques and concepts, are all important in intellectually understanding meditation.

There can be numerous scholarly studies conducted and statistics drawn up about meditation. There may even exist much research and data showing the benefits of a daily practice. However, without application, knowledge remains abstract.

After learning about navigation and sailing, you have to set sail to get anywhere. Similarly, someone who remains in a constant mode of seeking information, continuously jumping from one set of knowledge to another without attempting to apply it in their life, can never spiritually grow. No matter how much they learn, it is not enough to satiate their curiosity and appetite.

While it is important to open yourself up to intellectual study, real spiritual understanding occurs through implementation of what is read in books. At some point, one has to start putting into practice what has been learned. Education on any subject does nothing to change a human being if it does not in some way shift a person's thinking and add value to their life. The same is true with meditation.

One cannot solely study meditation from a book or debate about whether it works and expect to witness a change in behavior. Only allowing knowledge to sit in the mind will not rehabilitate thoughts and bring one closer to their higher nature. No amount of academic learning can compare to the deeper understanding one acquires through one's own experience.

Meditation cannot be understood without practice. The insights that one gains through meditation brings about internal changes in a way that mere reading cannot do. Only with a disciplined meditation practice can an individual come to the same realizations they are learning about in the writings of spiritual masters and gurus. When knowledge matures through practice it becomes wisdom. This is the only way theoretical understanding becomes a lived experience.

Ancient knowledge is meant to be adapted to modern

times. It exists for the purpose of implementing it into daily living without losing the true meaning and purpose behind it. Whatever is learned should be reflected upon and tried out. Seeing if and how it works, taking what is relevant, discarding that which is not helpful, these are the correct methods of incorporating spiritual teachings.

Once knowledge becomes a personal experience, spiritual books lose significance. One's own realizations are enough proof. They do not have to be read in a book. What once were intellectual concepts becomes a part of an individual's personality and character. Abstract philosophies become understood through direct experience. Words no longer hold the importance in understanding meditation that they once did. One becomes less concerned about things like labels and definitions. When a person is already living the knowledge in day-to-day life, what need do they have for descriptions and explanations? No words can describe what one is already realizing through their own experiences.

In meditation, we are moving from the mind to the heart, from thoughts to feeling. It is for this reason that meditation cannot be understood by logic alone; it must be realized through direct experience.

KEY VEDIC CONCEPTS: *Jnyana, Mananam, Nididhyasana, Shravanam, Vijnyana*

1.12 NOT REFLECTION AND CONTEMPLATION.

Meditation is not a passive activity. It is not the time to allow the mind to think whatever it wants indefinitely. Neither is meditation an opportunity to reflect on the past or set goals for the future. It is also not a chance to review the day or plan what chores need to be completed.

A person should not mistakenly believe they are meditating when they let the mind get carried away in different thoughts, memories, and fantasies. Nor should one take repressed emotions arising, such as crying or anger, to mean they are deeply meditating. Even pondering spiritual knowledge does not constitute meditation.

Thinking about our duties and obligations during meditation does not help us withdraw from the outside world. Creating life plans while attempting to meditate does not help us overcome desires and attachment to the individual consciousness. Contemplating sacred texts in meditation does not allow us to transcend thoughts.

In meditation, we are attempting to gain control over the mind. Allowing the mind to wander goes against this very intention. Rather, we are attempting to keep the mind focused on itself. We are practicing slowly reducing the quantity of thoughts, so that we can eventually make the mind quiet. Meditation can be thought of as continued self-efforts to discipline the mind. This cannot happen when focus goes outside of the self.

Reflection and contemplation are necessary parts of spiritual growth. This cannot be denied or underestimated. They are critical to removing the internal barriers that are preventing an individual from realizing their higher nature. A person has to understand why they see themselves as a limited being and continuously take action toward freeing themselves of self-imposed restrictions. One *should* be contemplating higher knowledge. A person *should* be attempting to understand and synthesize spiritual material into their life. *However,* reflection and contemplation do not constitute meditation. Instead, one should be supplementing their practice with self-study and introspection outside of meditation.

KEY VEDIC CONCEPTS: *Nigraha, Niruddha, Samyama*

1.13 DOES NOT PREVENT OR SOLVE ALL PROBLEMS.

Meditation does not eliminate all of life's problems and challenges. Things will not suddenly become perfect. Unfortunately, meditators are not absolved of the realities of life. Every one of us encounters ups and downs. As long as we are alive, we will experience circumstances beyond our control and the emotions that go along with it.

Daily meditation allows us to better cope with hardships and frustrations instead of suffering because of them. It helps us to positively manage the inevitable experiences of life. An everyday practice enables us to get to the root of problems and focus on the solutions. Meditation shifts the mindset to one of thoughtfully responding, rather than reacting out of habit.

Every day we have a choice in how we will meet the world. By regularly turning the mind toward the self in meditation, we begin to inquire into our thoughts and behaviors in the rest of our life. Am I going to dwell in the feelings of negativity, anger, sadness, jealousy, or fear over something I thought was going to happen in a certain way, but it didn't? Am I going to let it affect my self-worth, confidence, and ability to rise above mundane thinking?

A daily practice helps us to live peacefully with

ourselves. It does not stop the inconveniences in life or the happening of unexpected events. Neither does it prevent us from performing our obligations and responsibilities. As long as we choose to be active members of society, we will experience disappointments and frustrations. These are permanent fixtures of life that will never go away.

Meditation develops our ability to maintain right contact with the world, meaning without letting emotions overpower the mind. It helps us to become discerning over thoughts and cultivate an optimistic attitude. These qualities enable us to navigate our lives with calmness and ease no matter the external situation. So, as the activity of the world continues on around us, we remain ever equanimous.

KEY VEDIC CONCEPTS: *Sthirata, Sthir-mati, Sthitaprajna*

1.14 DOES NOT MEAN DEPRIVING YOURSELF.

In the beginning, sustaining a daily meditation habit may be difficult. There will exist the practical challenges of balancing responsibilities with trying to develop an everyday meditation practice.

Additionally, learning a meditation technique suited to an individual's personality and temperament may take experimenting. Continued efforts will be required. Even during meditation, uneasiness may be felt in maintaining a comfortable seated posture. One may have difficulty in keeping the mind from wandering. After all, the nature of the human mind is not to dwell in itself and be still. We rather ruminate in fanciful thinking and go after objects of immediate gratification. These are all common hurdles that many people experience and they can be overcome with a steady practice.

Moreover, some people approach meditation as a type of punishment. They believe it needs to be something forced upon themselves because it is good for their health, like going on a diet for the body. Sometimes this leads to meditating with a pessimistic attitude. They may feel that they just want to get their meditation over with and done. But, this type of mindset cannot create any meaningful change within a person.

Also, some people create fear in their mind that prevents them from meditating. Scared of emotions that may arise or having to possibly face past hurts creates an immediate roadblock. The anticipation of potentially letting go of certain people or situations stops a person from even trying to meditate.

Daily meditation does not mean depriving oneself. Some people falsely believe that meditation should be a rigid compulsion. They assume meditation requires renouncing sensory engagement, living an ascetic life, or blindly following a religious code of conduct that is neither understood intellectually, nor spiritually.

A person should not view sitting in meditation as a challenge to see how long one can endure the pain. Neither should creating a daily meditation practice mean giving up necessities and obligations. Suppressing natural tendencies only results in greater harm to an individual. One should not deny their desires and inherent needs. Trying to sustain an everyday meditation habit should never feel like punishment.

This is why it is important to cultivate a long-term, daily meditation practice. One should naturally come to a point where reducing desires is not seen as a sacrifice, but rather a natural outcome of one's inner development.

With time, an individual organically removes excess and lives with less.

If today you thought about changing careers to a new field, without absolutely any previous training, of course you would feel overwhelmed and perhaps even scared. You may be filled with doubt thinking about the years of training ahead of you. But, like any professional endeavor, it takes our own efforts to gain the knowledge and experience. Once you are thoroughly prepared, you no longer have the same fear that plagued your mind when you began the journey.

Similarly, meditation requires preparation and consistency. One slowly evolves into a different person. Whatever is meant to arise in your mind, happens for a reason. You have to be cleansed of emotions, attachments, and ego so that you can elevate your mind to a higher consciousness. One has to steadily lead the mind to quietude. This evolution happens as a result of continual inner work, not because of self-coercion.

One should develop such devotion to their practice that they are drawn to sitting every day without resistance or doubt. Meditation should happen out of willingness. It is this enthusiasm that helps someone to keep going even when challenges arise. Initially, what takes conscious effort becomes something a person wants to do out of realizing the benefits of meditation for themselves.

Some people think, *How can I be happy when others are suffering?* I will not allow myself to be at peace because this world is a miserable place full of hate and violence. However, when one focuses on shortcomings, they are not only doing themselves a disservice, but they are also depriving humanity of the light they can shine on others. Living in the lower mind, negative thinking, defaulting to instinctive reactions, does not help the world. You have to lift yourself up, by yourself, only then can you inspire others to do the same for themselves.

KEY VEDIC CONCEPTS: *Aparigraha, Pratyaya, Prayatna, Sadhana, Shanti*

1.15 NOT SELFISH.

Oftentimes meditation is seen as a selfish pursuit. The insights and realizations taking place within a person cannot be seen by anyone else. When others cannot witness the inner work or they are not a part of it, there is a tendency to dismiss it as self-absorbed or unimportant.

However, meditation demands and requires that it be practiced in solitude. Daily meditation significantly improves not only the way someone responds to the world, but also how they interact with it. Meditating every day helps a person develop more restraint over thoughts and thus, makes the mind peaceful. Such an individual fulfills obligations and carries out responsibilities with a positive mindset. Remaining ever present, one moves through one's daily life with calmness and balance.

Having realized inner tranquility within oneself naturally makes a person feel like sharing their experience with others. Showing people that they too can rise out of their own suffering through their own lived experience of it gives others the much needed hope and confidence to begin their own inner journeys.

In this way, the path toward self-knowledge and expanded awareness is not selfish. Meditation actually changes a person from being only concerned about their own well-being to considering the wellness of the entire community.

Even some of those who have become enlightened through their own self-efforts do not completely abandon the world. Many swamis and sages write books and give spiritual talks. They share their knowledge selflessly for the betterment of society. They become guides for others by living as an example of the human potential. We should look up to them with aspiration for our own internal possibilities.

Living in equanimity does not mean we stop trying to improve our surroundings. If anything, daily meditation builds our conviction of purpose. We no longer only think and work toward our own advantage, but think about how to improve the situation of all individuals, in the family and society at large.

Although meditation is practiced in isolation, the benefits of it go beyond the self. Aim to lift people out of their low vibrations by raising your own, do not meet them there. By living in higher consciousness within yourself, you are spreading light to others. What nobler service to perform in this world than to realize your own blissful nature.

KEY VEDIC CONCEPTS: *Prasanna, Shanti*

1.16 MATERIAL KNOWLEDGE IS NOT SPIRITUAL KNOWLEDGE.

What we learn in school to help us earn a living, the education we receive toward obtaining a professional degree, and the academic books we study, all constitute material knowledge. We apply these skills to become financially prosperous and create a comfortable lifestyle. Material knowledge is important for survival in this world. However, it does nothing to recondition the mind.

Spiritual knowledge discovered through the inner realizations of sages in the past compose the philosophies that we now read about in books. These sacred texts set forth principles and elucidate practical applications for higher living. They ignite a spark within us toward living in a high-minded way. They help us set noble goals. These teachings provide the roadmap toward realizing eternal peace and ultimate happiness.

It is due to the experiences of those who have walked this path before us that we know purifying the self of anger, lust, greed, and jealousy is necessary for making the mind stable and quiet. It is from their insights that we have guidance on how to undo patterns of the conditioned mind in order to gain control over the senses.

It is this ancient wisdom that shows us how to slowly overcome our material desires and attachments, so that we can realize inner freedom. It is through application of these practices that self-knowledge unfolds and leads us to realize absolute bliss.

Material knowledge improves our lives, but not in the same way. Only spiritual knowledge helps us live in this world happily and peacefully by creating a fundamental change from within. Together, like the two wings of a bird, material and spiritual knowledge are important to living a healthy and thriving life.

KEY VEDIC CONCEPTS: *Kshetra, Kshetrajnya*

1.17 SPIRITUAL KNOWLEDGE MUST NOT ONLY BE STUDIED, BUT ALSO LIVED.

This is one of the most important sutras in the book. Many people consider someone who has read scriptures to be spiritual. However, even a person who has memorized an entire canon of religious texts still only has an intellectual understanding of these readings. Someone who focuses merely on being able to debate the nuanced interpretations of holy books lacks the personal experience of this knowledge. Living spiritually does not *only* mean saying prayers and chanting, reading religious books, or conducting rituals. Nor does it mean to solely quote sacred writings, perfect mantras, or learn how to creatively narrate moral tales.

It is absolutely necessary for a person to increase self-understanding through the reading of sacred texts and spiritual literature. One *should* educate oneself through the different means available, such as watching videos, participating in group discussions, and attending talks by spiritual masters. *However,* it should not stop there. One then needs to go further and make attempts to integrate this knowledge into one's life. Spiritual knowledge has to be directly experienced in order for it to transform the mind.

Taking time to think about and absorb what has been read and seeing if and how it applies, are the first steps to practicing these higher ideals. While a person contemplates on what they have learned, they should simultaneously be engaging in self-study and daily meditation. This helps one to determine which concepts and ideas are useful for their individual growth.

Attempts should then be made to incorporate relevant teachings and putting into action any realizations experienced through meditation. This progression in thinking and behavior gradually changes a person from the inside out. Slowly, spiritual knowledge goes from being abstract to becoming a part of one's character.

A true spiritual practice means accepting the circumstances that are unfolding before you with equanimity of mind, while performing your duties to the best of your abilities. This includes maintaining patience, avoiding preconceptions and assumptions of others, having self-awareness, and choosing to respond instead of react. We practice spirituality by developing the ability to spontaneously evaluate feelings as they are occurring, continuously reflecting, and understanding our defaults and finding ways to self-correct.

Living spiritual knowledge means that every day you are attempting to understand your inner nature, learn from your defects, enhance your noble qualities, and better yourself through continuous self-reflection and inner study. An individual who makes consistent efforts to apply what they are learning will eventually uncover the soul-infinite bliss within.

KEY VEDIC CONCEPTS: *Mananam, Nididhyasana, Shravanam, Svadhyaya*

1.18 REAL SPIRITUAL PROGRESS CAN ONLY BE OBSERVED FROM WITHIN.

The real changes from meditation occur in the mind. No one else can be a witness to what goes on there other than you. For this reason, they can only be observed from within.

Your meditation progress will not be wholly visible to others. If we think about it objectively, we also cannot completely witness someone else's personal growth. We cannot see how much courage it is taking someone to face a certain challenge. We are unable to tell just by looking at someone how much patience they are trying to cultivate in dealing with a matter. We cannot perceive how someone is trying to overcome their own misconceptions and judgments. We may have no idea of the personal tests a person may be enduring on a daily basis. Therefore, we can never fully comprehend the magnitude of inner strength it is taking for someone to move beyond their own limitations.

Similarly, you cannot show others how far you have come on your path. What you derive from meditation will not *always* be tangible to other people. Although others may notice changes in your behavior, the continuous internal work you are doing to overcome certain thoughts patterns or to accept the root causes of your agitations are not always observable to those around you. They cannot be brought out and presented like some material object. Other people will never likely see the complete breadth of ongoing changes taking place inside of you.

Neither will you be able to create or control situations to show the results of your meditation practice. We are tested each day in unforeseeable ways. When your own mind is unpredictable to you, even you may not know how you will respond to a particular circumstance.

Sometimes, we feel the need to display to others through outward appearance just how spiritual we are by emphasizing the number of followers we have or by the kinds of clothes we wear. Even though our inner life is a mess and we are struggling with our own mind, we continue quoting spiritual people and philosophy and presenting it as our personal practice.

Spirituality is not a show. It is not an ego-boosting endeavor. In fact, those things are barriers to progress. They are the antithesis of why we have a daily practice. Meditation should be practiced to remove these hindrances so that one becomes free from the confines of the mind and moves towards liberation.

Unfortunately, very few people, if any, will value your meditation practice. Most are too focused on worldly pursuits to appreciate your spiritual growth. Some may even mistake your commitment to meditation with being a pushover, a simpleton, naive, confused, or even misled. The primary motivation should never be validation; rather, a real spiritual seeker gets inspired by gaining peace of mind, not the expectation of accolades. The important thing is that you value your meditation practice.

One has to have a bigger purpose, a noble ideal to work toward in meditation. Someone who has set their sights higher can never be stopped from personal growth. The true meditation aspirant puts in the time and effort, maintains self-discipline, while remaining flexible, positive, and willing to learn about themselves. Persistently making attempts to understand where you are in need of improvement through self-reflection and quietly adjusting behavior without seeking attention are the markers of spiritual progress. Peace of mind comes from continuously doing the inner work. Slowing down, responding with evenness of mind, and selflessness are natural outcomes of daily meditation, not because you are forcing yourself to behave this way.

KEY VEDIC CONCEPTS: *Ishta Devata, Jnyana, Sadhaka*

CHAPTER 2

Preparing the Mind

2.1 BASIC NEEDS MUST BE MET.

A mind occupied with how to meet basic human needs cannot think about meditation. There can be no energy to give to spiritual pursuits when a person's primary concerns are hunger, shelter, sleep, warmth, and safety. When all thoughts are focused on how one will survive each day, attention cannot be directed to higher thinking.

Taking care of one's essential needs comes first and foremost. A person should not neglect them or think they are selfish. Meditation should never come at the price of one's own well-being. It should not be that someone skips a meal or sacrifices sleep in order to meditate every day. Depriving oneself in this way is neither healthy nor sustainable.

Meditation is a conscious activity that requires physical and mental energy. It is an active practice that calls for sitting upright, consciously directing the mind, and developing concentration. Additionally, sitting every day requires stamina and willpower. One has to maintain the health of the body because the body is a vehicle to realizing the higher nature. If the body is sick, weak, or tired, it cannot sit in regular meditation. Focusing and quieting the mind demands that the body first be in good condition. So, it is important to keep fit through diet and exercise. This helps us to properly use our energy toward elevating the mind.

One should be mindful of the quantity and quality of food eaten. Overeating makes a person feel lethargic and creates dullness in the mind. However, not eating enough makes one easily fatigued. A person should also receive adequate amounts of sleep, meaning not too much or too little. Oversleeping makes one feel lazy and unmotivated, whereas not having enough sleep makes it challenging to remain focused. Moreover, one should make sure hygiene is taken care of and that everyday bodily needs such as brushing teeth and bathing are fulfilled.

These are all prerequisites to sustaining an everyday meditation practice. Not only should these basic necessities not be neglected, but there should also be a proper balance of them in one's life. Only once these needs are met and maintained, can a person direct their energy towards meditation.

KEY VEDIC CONCEPTS: *Mitaahara, Svapnavabodhasya, Yuktahara*

2.2 DUTIES AND OBLIGATIONS SHOULD CONTINUE TO BE PERFORMED.

Having a daily meditation practice does not mean giving up commitments that we have made in this world. Providing for family members that are dependent on our physical and emotional support should be maintained. Contributing to society through hard work and efforts should not be abandoned. Giving back to the community for the opportunities and privileges we have been given should also continue with enthusiastic spirit.

In addition, we shouldn't pessimistically approach our duties just because they cannot be avoided. It is our attitude toward our obligations that needs to continuously be checked and refined. Performing our actions with the mindset that we are helping to bring joy into others' lives and thus, decreasing their suffering, brings about a healthy integration of fulfilling our duties and leading a spiritual life.

Sustaining such a selfless attitude does not come without changing our thinking. Sometimes we may feel that it would be easier to give up all of our commitments than shift our perspective and change the way we approach our work. However, physically giving up our attachments means nothing if we still desire and crave the comforts they provide. Renunciation happens in the mind, not merely through physical action.

Instead, we should aim to do our work by removing attachment to the anxiety of the results of our actions. The mind becomes disturbed in the process of performing any activity when it focuses on the quality of an outcome. A person cannot work efficiently worrying about whether what they are doing will yield the kind of result they expect. The work suffers; instead of concentrating on the task, one becomes consumed with thoughts of the kind of reaction it will produce. Wondering whether it will be appreciated or criticized, a person cannot let go of how they will be affected.

Whether a person works by keeping the result of an action in mind or not, there will be some kind of outcome. It cannot be that a cause will have no effect. Although we cannot control the type of result an action produces, we do have power over how we perform our duties. Only when one can develop the ability to give wholeheartedly, without any kind of expectation, can inner happiness be found. A person gives their best in any activity when they do not focus on what they will gain from it.

Instead, one should do their level best to keep their mind on something noble, whether that is God or the higher self. When the focus becomes larger than the self, personal agendas and selfish motives automatically drop away. When we dedicate our actions in service to something bigger than ourselves, we perform our duties selflessly. When we cultivate the understanding that the divine is in everyone and everything, our actions no longer become just about ourselves. Emotions no longer overpower evenness of mind. We approach our work with calmness, instead of excitement. As a result, we are more efficient and productive. Our daily work becomes rewarding and enriching.

Naturally, one may find it challenging to balance daily meditation with obligations and leisurely activities. Usually, people let go of their meditation practice because time becomes a factor in sitting every day. But, this is a mistake. Instead, of prioritizing meditation, they leave it and make everything else important. Giving up meditation, the very thing that can ultimately lead to real happiness, should not be relinquished. Instead, the other things that are used as a way to fill up time should slowly be let go.

This naturally happens as one progresses in meditation. An individual may find that certain activities are no longer appealing or some relationships do not provide the same fulfillment. A person should not stop contemplating on what serves their higher goal and finding rational, well-thought-out courses of action.

This is all to say that one should continue carrying out their duties and responsibilities. At the same time, a person should regularly assess what is necessary and unnecessary to their self-development, while maintaining the energy needed for daily meditation.

KEY VEDIC CONCEPTS: *Dwesha, Karma Yoga, Raga, Vairagya, Viveka*

2.3 KEEP THE SAME ROUTINE.

Keeping the same routine every day helps to maintain a meditation practice. It is only with regularity that one can make any kind of progress in meditation. A person should follow a daily schedule, manage time efficiently, and properly plan the day, so that meditation does not get left out amidst other obligations and responsibilities.

When one's routine gets interrupted, it becomes challenging to keep a consistent meditation practice. This includes not only meditating at the same time every day, but also maintaining the duration and level of concentration one has developed up until that point. Additionally, being able to sit comfortably in the same seated posture and getting used to a meditation technique requires repetition over a period of time.

As is common, many people approach meditation very enthusiastically in the beginning. However, their eagerness fades when they realize that one needs to keep applying the same effort and methods over time to create a true change in consciousness.

This should not serve to discourage, but rather help a person realize that transformation is within their grasp. One has the potential to determine their own fate by slowly rehabilitating the mind and changing how they experience the world.

When an irregular schedule cannot be avoided, necessary adjustments should be well-thought-out in advance so one does not miss the opportunity to meditate in the day. Meditating for shorter periods, at a different time in the day than usual, or creating a makeshift space to sit for meditation are strategies one should mindfully think through under varied circumstances.

Although these methods could be applied during unpredictable times, they should not become a habit. The ideal is to continue practicing the same meditation routine, meaning the method and duration that one has developed, in the same place.

Routines and schedules will naturally change with the different phases of life. This sutra should not be read to mean that someone should always remain the same without wanting to evolve and grow. Rather, this sutra should inspire in one the intentionality of daily living and spark a thoughtful and purposeful meditation practice.

KEY VEDIC CONCEPTS: *Nigraha, Niyama*

2.4 ENVIRONMENT HAS TO INTENTIONALLY BE CREATED.

Considering that we cannot always be surrounded by the optimal environment for meditation, we have to intentionally create it. We want to cultivate such a space that the mind will be able to focus on itself. Since much of our time is spent inside of the home and it is usually the place where a person meditates, it has one of the biggest influences on our daily practice. The home environment affects our physical energy and capacity for higher thinking. Our thoughts either grow or shrink according to our surroundings. If we want to enhance the effects of meditation, such as positive thinking, expanded awareness, and an elevated mind, the atmosphere in the home should help nurture this inner development.

The place where we live sets up our mindset for the day and determines how we will interact with the world. If we surround ourselves with clutter and allow negative energy inside our homes, disharmony will pervade other aspects of our lives. Instead, if we are conscious of what we allow inside the home, from material items to people whose energies remain behind in our spaces, we will practice the same discrimination in the rest of our lives. We begin creating this self-discipline through our immediate environment.

Inside the home one carries out the basic human activities required for health and hygiene. The areas in which these activities are being done should be kept clean. The place you eat should be free from dust. The food we put into our bodies not only gives us physical energy, but its ingredients give us the fuel for our thoughts. Wherever food is being cooked or stored inside the home should be clean.

The place you sleep should be free from clutter. Our beds contain accumulated energy from each day. We leave our imprints in our bedsheets and on our pillows by the thoughts and dreams we have there every night. The place where you bathe should be sanitary and clean. Here, we purify ourselves every day.

Where we spend the most time has a profound impact on our well-being and thoughts. Ideally, home should be a place that encourages a steady practice. Our space should create the right conditions for the effects of our meditations to be realized. The way we keep our home is a reflection of our state of mind, while the items we keep inside the home represent the quality of our thoughts.

What types of objects are in your space? What do they say about your values and standard of life? Do they help you feel free or restricted? This self-evaluation is not about materialism, rather it's a reflection of our attitudes and principles. When the home is clean, uplifting, and peaceful, the mind will be the same.

Even if a person is not using their home for meditation, these same principles apply to whichever space is being utilized for a daily practice. It should be clean and clutter free, as well as intentionally created to support higher contemplation and quiet inward reflection.

KEY VEDIC CONCEPTS: *Aparigraha, Desha, Saucha*

2.5 CREATE A MEDITATION ALTAR.

An altar gives us a dedicated place to meditate. Other spaces in the home utilized for meditation cannot evoke the same feeling and devotion as a designated area. If a person is meditating in the same place as they are sleeping or eating, it will not only be distracting, but can discourage a sustained meditation practice. Having a specific place that one intentionally goes to only for meditation, outside of other activities, helps develop a consistent practice.

The place where you meditate should be free from odor, clutter, and dust. The area should be well ventilated, with enough fresh air to prevent distraction and discomfort. You should be able to access the altar whenever the feeling to meditate arises and especially during the fixed time you have committed to practicing every day.

Ideally, the altar should be in a quiet and private area. Depending on the space available in the home, it can be placed in the corner of a room or an empty counter or shelf. If no space restrictions exist, then an entire room designated for meditation would help provide the solitude and calming atmosphere needed to go inward.

A person should personalize the space with elements from nature, calming scents, statues or photos of deities, or anything else that helps invoke a light and vibrant feeling within oneself. Any rituals in preparation for sitting, such as lighting a candle or burning incense, also help to indicate to the mind that it is time to meditate. All of these elements improve the chances of a person maintaining a daily meditation practice over a period of time.

Not only will a meditation altar enhance a practice, it will also motivate you when time seems limited or enthusiasm diminishes. Through consistent use of the space, a positive and inviting energy gets created there, organically drawing one in to connect with the higher self. The altar begins to naturally attract one to sit and meditate.

There are certain places that have a powerful influence on us. By merely being in them we feel an incredible and profound connection to the universal spirit. Walking through a holy city, being inside a place of worship, or sitting outside in nature, can immediately bring us immense peace. One should aim to create that same free and uplifting feeling not only inside the home, but also within oneself.

Your meditation altar is essentially the temple you have in your home. It not only provides a designated space for your practice that inspires you to sit every day, but it is also a powerful way to incorporate spirituality into your daily life. The space serves as a reminder to live in elevated consciousness and transcend limited beliefs. It should help create in you a reverential feeling toward a higher ideal and direct your mind to rise above mundane thinking. A sacred space can be the catalyst we need to create a change from within.

KEY VEDIC CONCEPTS: *Shuddha*

2.6 USE YOUR MEDITATION ALTAR.

Once you have created a meditation altar, you have to actually use it. This seems obvious, but oftentimes the excitement of creating a sacred space overshadows the fact that one will actually be sitting and using it every day.

In the beginning, you may have to make intentional and continuous efforts to sit at your altar. This is why it is important to personalize your meditation area according to your needs and tastes. Your sacred space should naturally draw you in with elements that make you feel peaceful and relaxed. However, an altar should not just become part of the home decor, as something to show others when they visit. Neither should it be used to put your spirituality on display.

Buying items and designing a space are done for the purpose of utilizing it to sit in higher contemplation and turning the mind toward the self. It would be unfortunate to create such an inviting and uplifting area only for it to never be used. It is akin to cooking an elaborate meal with many courses and never eating it. After making the effort and putting in the time to create a meditation altar, it should be engaged with every day.

Usually, as a person maintains a daily practice, they

start to notice the benefits of having a designated area and witness the improvements within themselves. Gradually, having a meditation altar becomes less about the items kept there and how it looks, and more about one's inner growth. Slowly, one no longer has to make conscious attempts at sitting every day because the changes they see inside of themselves naturally motivate them to meditate. In this way, a meditation altar is a tool for withdrawing the mind from the outer world and going inward. It helps in creating a daily habit. Having a meditation space is just a step on the journey to the self, not the final destination.

KEY VEDIC CONCEPTS: *Dhyana, Niyamit*

2.7 ENVIRONMENT EXTENDS BEYOND PHYSICAL SPACE.

Whether we realize it or not, how we engage our senses creates our environment as much as our physical surroundings. What we feed the mind leaves subtle and lasting impressions. The images we expose ourselves to, what we listen to, the language we use, the work we do, what we eat, how we spend our time, what we prioritize, how we use our energy, all form the basis of our individual consciousness.

The various outside engagements we occupy ourselves with and the different ways we interact with the world affects the stability of our minds. We have to be careful to not surround ourselves with things that could easily pull us down to a lower state of mind. The moment you come on the Internet, the potential for comparisons, judgments, and jealousy begins. The moment you turn on the television, the potential for lust, materialism, fear, and self-doubt begins. The moment you step outside of your home and interact with others, the potential for greed, anger, and envy begins. Our perceptions influence our thinking and reasoning in everyday life. These impressions form the way we see the world and each other.

As long as we are living in this body, we are vulnerable to external conditions creating internal agitations. Because we will never be absolved of the continuous experiences of life that have the possibility of producing further attachments and desires, we should try our best to improve our mental condition. A disturbed mind full of emotions, such as anger, jealousy, and passion, needs to first become calm in order to be able to meditate. It is only a stable mind that can focus. This becomes difficult to do when one voluntarily engages the senses in thoughtless preoccupations and passively accepts external stimuli. This does not mean that a person should shut themselves off from outside engagements. Rather, it requires that one exhibit more control over their environment.

Unfortunately, we are increasingly living in a world where our experiences are managed for us. We do not have as much control over what images and messages we are exposed to as modern conveniences and technological advances become more a part of daily life. Although this makes it more challenging for one to be selective of the quality of content they are exposed to, it does not prevent one from being intentional in designing positive experiences for oneself.

We should create such an atmosphere around us that our thoughts remain pure and our minds stay elevated.

Listening to inspiring words, reading uplifting material, looking at serene images, sharing knowledge to help raise the minds of society (as opposed to gossiping), engaging in activities that make one feel hopeful and productive, eating healthy food, and keeping positive company are all things one can intentionally work toward incorporating more often in their lives.

The people we choose to surround ourselves with regularly should inspire our continued inner growth. We should feel encouraged by them to put into practice our spiritual readings and the effects of our meditation practice. We should remain mindful of being around those who do not cause further negative impressions in the mind, but instead support us in moving toward self-unfoldment.

We should intentionally be creating the types of experiences that help us become more detached from the ego and leave positive imprints on the mind. Keeping the mind pure and elevated means consciously evaluating whether our activities are either helping us grow closer or farther away from realizing our divine nature. What we put into our minds affects us on the subtlest levels.

As we continue working on undoing our past impressions, we are simultaneously accumulating new experiences. These affect how we think of the past and create even newer impressions in the mind. As we determine how to interact with the world, we should try our best to choose experiences that do not further agitate the mind. The senses should be engaged in ways that help to uplift the consciousness, and move through the world with evenness and equanimity. Ideally, we want to keep our minds so high that where in the past we would have ruminated in conditioned thinking, we now have rehabilitated our thoughts such that these habitual patterns no longer get nurtured.

KEY VEDIC CONCEPTS: *Indriyas, Karma, Satsanga*

2.8 REAL HAPPINESS MEANS PEACE OF MIND.

When we say happiness, what we really want to experience is peace of mind. The two cannot be felt in isolation from one another.

Isn't it so that when you feel any happiness that you also feel a sense of peace? Even if it is temporary, happiness usually comes after an expectation is met or a goal has been achieved. When things go according to what we have imagined, we feel a sense of relief. One can use the many examples from their own life to see that happiness comes when the mind feels satisfied.

However, this happiness does not last for long because it relies on the outcome of some external happening. When the desire for a particular result remains unrealized, the individual response is generally with a wave of emotions. Anger, resentment, and disappointment take over the mind. A person loses the ability to think logically and rationally. Even when expectations are met, we still crave for more. As long as one keeps giving the power of their happiness to something outside of their control, the mind will be unbalanced, erratic, and fluctuating. The mind has to first be made quiet and stable to realize peace from within.

What stands in the way of peace of mind are jealousy, anger, passion, greed, lust, strong preferences for likes and dislikes, ego, rigid thinking, attachments, and expectations. Lasting happiness can only exist when outer circumstances no longer affect evenness of mind. Real happiness cannot be taken away by anything temporary and external.

Someone who has found real inner happiness has the ability to be alone and not feel lonely. They maintain control over their thoughts and have a restrained mind. They do not have extreme emotions and mood swings but rather maintain a balanced mind. They have the ability to accept a given situation for what it is instead of creating expectations for a certain outcome. They are not driven by ego but instead act out of the good for humankind. They continuously engage in self-inquiry, striving for simplicity and purity of thoughts.

It is impossible for one to be happy, unless they have found peace within themselves. Only when happiness does not depend on a circumstance, person, or thing, will true inner-lasting joy be realized.

We step onto the path of realizing inner peace through a daily meditation practice. Slowly, we work on letting go of our limitations as we come to experience our true, sublime nature. Through patience and persistence, we get closer to realizing true inner happiness.

KEY VEDIC CONCEPTS: *Kama, Krodha, Lobha, Mada, Matsarya, Moha, Samatva, Samyama, Santosha, Shad-ripu, Shanti*

2.9 PEACE OF MIND IS REALIZED BY PURIFYING THE MIND.

In this book, purifying the mind does not refer to cleaning a dirty mind full of vices, immoralities, and perversions. Neither does it mean removing evil thoughts or making amends for ill deeds, nor reforming the mind to follow religious doctrine out of fear of moral punishment. Purifying the mind means to become aware of unconscious habits and tendencies by making them conscious, while gradually eliminating their control over the mind, so that one can realize their own blissful nature.

All human beings dwell in different levels of thinking, whether those are memories, fantasies, imagination, desires, or recalling past situations. When one assumes these thoughts to be Reality, the mind becomes emotional with passion, lust, anger, jealousy, and greed. One's identity becomes defined by what one has experienced, thought, and felt. This becomes the lens through which one views and interacts with the world. As a result, a person comes to suffer from these self-created limitations and inadequacies. An individual needs to remove the veil of ignorance that has been created by identifying with these various thoughts and emotions.

The mind is impure due to the past impressions that have formed from life experiences. As long as the mind is occupied with the different forms of thought currents, it will not be able to recognize the higher nature. Gradually and patiently, a person should work toward ridding the mind of these impurities that have built up over time.

When the mind becomes free from the preoccupation of thoughts, it is able to be fully present. The mind no longer stays restricted in ruminating on thoughts of the past, excitement of the present, or worrying about the future. One can accept each moment as it is unfolding instead of projecting judgments and expectations. Through this process, the mind becomes calm, alert, and ripe to abide in the self.

KEY VEDIC CONCEPTS: *Chitta, Shuddha, Vasanas, Vikalpa*

2.10 PURIFY THE MIND BY REMOVING DOUBTS AND DEVELOPING FAITH.

For meditation to have any effect, the mind must first be prepared to receive inner knowledge. If one skeptically begins a practice, then meditation has no chance of having any positive outcome. When someone is focused on discrediting and challenging meditation, the mind becomes preoccupied with finding something wrong with it. A person consumed with questioning in order to unveil a flaw or learning with the intent to find fault is looking for a reason to not meditate. Higher knowledge will never dawn in a person who has made their mind up to never accept it.

An individual who adamantly believes that meditation will not work without even trying it or gives up on it after a short time will make very little progress. Someone who engages in constant intellectual debate and demands proof that meditation works, relies on external means to gain internal understanding. This approach will never remove doubt and build faith.

This is not to say that a healthy type of questioning must not exist. To take up any practice on blind faith is foolish. Unless doubts are cleared, they will inevitably keep rising. New knowledge cannot enter the mind of a person filled with uncertainty, judgment, and questioning. One has to first break free from their own resistance for meditation to take place. The mind has to be ready to receive the insights that come with a daily meditation practice.

Often a person will find a meditation technique that works, practice it for a few days, and then do away with it after finding some flaw in it. This happens not because the benefit of the tool has changed, but because the mind has created a reason to no longer make an effort. In this instance, it is the mind that needs to be fixed, not the meditation method.

Similarly, when one doubts spiritual knowledge, it indicates that one needs to look deep within oneself to uncover their own self-created barriers. A person has to be willing to learn through their own understanding. Instead of following along blindly because someone has told them that meditation leads to lasting happiness, one must be available to realize it through their own self-efforts. First-hand experience removes resistance and strengthens the intellect to keep going. Faith will be the natural outcome of one's direct experience. It will be faith that keeps a person motivated and committed to a daily meditation practice.

Sometimes one will hear of other people having a vision of the divine or seeing an image of God form in natural surroundings, such as on a stone or on the bark of a tree. Often the validity of these sightings are doubted. But, why does it bother us? Questioning and dismissing it says something about our own faith. That someone has such faith in their ideal and upholds it with such high regard that they see it in everything and everywhere, is the height of devotion we should be trying to attain within ourselves.

You *should* see the divine in everything, in every person, object, and situation. The higher self should always be with you. We ourselves do not have faith and doubt others when they do. The devotion in others should make you question your own instead of suspecting it!

Devotion develops when the mind focuses on a higher ideal. Continuously attempting to bring one-pointed focus to an image or symbol of God or the higher self during meditation changes the direction of thought flow. Quality of thoughts improve upon contemplation on the auspicious. The mind slowly rises to meet an elevated vision. An individual starts living with a deeper purpose when aspirations become noble. Devotion removes doubt through a deeply instilled and unshakable faith.

One needs to constantly be working on overcoming

one's own struggles, deficiencies, and inadequacies. Whatever you feel is lacking in you, realize this is not your true nature. Verify what you are learning about meditation and spirituality through your own lived experience of it. Understand the outcome of your life lies in your own hands. By slowly developing a strong will and determination, doubt will naturally go away and be replaced with firm faith.

KEY VEDIC CONCEPTS: *Bhakti Yoga, Shraddha*

2.11 PURIFY THE MIND BY REGULATING THE SENSES.

The mind determines what to look at with the eyes, what to listen to with the ears, what to taste with the mouth, what to touch with the skin, and what to smell with the nose. Unfortunately, the majority of people are not in control of their senses. Instead of the mind directing the movement of the senses, the senses lead the mind. Whatever stimulates the tastebuds, excites the eyes, and arouses the nose, ears, and skin, one goes after without restraint.

When we find something pleasurable, we want more of it. Often when we keep returning for the same experience, either we do not derive similar pleasure or our happiness becomes exhausted from that one object. We crave to have that same satisfied feeling again. We seek other means, this time through new sense activities. As this cycle continues, one relinquishes more control over the senses and gives up the ability to guide them.

The mind is an enemy to those who follow the whims of the senses. It is only when thoughts become restrained that they can purposefully be guided to direct the senses. A mind sure of itself has mastery over the senses. One chooses where to bring their attention and what to focus on. A person develops mindful contact with objects and prevents overindulgence. One who has gained control over their senses does not easily become influenced by external objects, and therefore maintains a balanced mind. An unyielding mind discerns between outside engagements that create negative and positive impressions. As a result, one understands limitations, makes healthier decisions, and has self-control.

Additionally, when a person frees themselves from the preoccupation of sense activities this creates space in the mind for higher thinking. Finite energy not being consumed in uncontrollably running after outside pleasures can be directed toward inner development. There is enough energy to utilize toward higher contemplation and superior activities.

An unwavering mind engages the senses in useful and productive ways that help to expand the consciousness. Ideally, our sense organs are meant to be used toward making the mind peaceful, increasing self-awareness, and elevating thoughts, so that we can move toward liberation. This is a privilege given to us as human beings, which other animals are not gifted with. An individual with self-discipline over the sense organs keeps their mind in the higher consciousness as they navigate through this world. The mind is a friend to the person whose higher self is constantly available to them through control of the senses.

A person should naturally come to the realization that overdoing in sense pleasures takes one away from knowing real peace. It is only with direct experience that one realizes how aimless engrossments with the outer world only temporarily relieve the mind before it again goes in search of happiness. Organically, an individual should develop self-control and regulation over the mind. Daily meditation helps one through this step-by-step process by steadily gaining restraint over the sense organs and naturally reaching a place of equanimity.

This sutra should not mistakenly be read to mean that one should stop all sense enjoyments. Instead, one should engage in external activities through a firm mind, so that energy does not get unnecessarily used in indulging in the senses and taking vitality away from inner contemplation.

KEY VEDIC CONCEPTS: *Abhyasa, Dama, Indriyas, Samyama, Shama, Vairagya, Viveka*

2.12 PURIFY THE MIND BY DEVELOPING A BALANCED AND STEADY MIND.

When you are angry and someone tries to speak sense to you, do you listen? No, you are overcome by your emotions. Your mind is not available to you. You first have to come back to a calmer state before you can objectively assess the situation and determine the right course of action.

A person who allows emotions to overpower them gives up the ability to intelligently interact with the world. It cannot be possible to make rational decisions when judgment has been suspended by jealousy, greed, anger, and passion. One loses the capacity to think logically.

An oscillating mind is a victim of emotions. It quickly reacts and becomes disturbed by simple things. When the mind is fickle, it gets easily swayed and distressed. Mood and behavior become determined by external circumstances. Such a person has very little control over their mind. They behave out of impulse and reaction. The mind cannot be quiet when it is constantly vulnerable to external influences.

A natural result of daily meditation is a balanced

mind. Living in a higher consciousness means transcending fear, worry, and stress, those things that weigh us down and make us react out of panic. Only when we can apply the higher mind to our everyday lives, can we make decisions that are healthy and bring out the best in us.

Balance of mind does not mean inaction. It means approaching each moment with thoughtfulness and practicality, raising the mindset to arrive at a solution. To see something clearly, one needs to become emotionally detached from it. Detachment should happen naturally, through a direct realization of it, not by repression or forceful denial.

Detachment does not mean physically renouncing the material world and abandoning all responsibilities. Detachment means realizing the temporariness of an object or situation and not allowing it to affect the balance of mind. It means forming the correct relationship with a person, situation, or object by understanding its purpose and place in one's life. Detachment means having restraint over thoughts instead of being influenced by conditioned patterns and previous experiences.

Being able to view something objectively requires that one not form an expectation of happiness from it. A person who recognizes that permanent joy cannot be derived from something outside of oneself lives with a balanced mind. External circumstances do not effect someone who navigates this world through an equanimous mind.

During the times one cannot maintain control over their environment, a steady mind naturally filters out what it needs to so that it can remain in a higher state. Such an individual remains even-minded, even in adverse situations.

A person with a balanced mind still loves, feels compassion, and expresses sentiment, but they are not overcome by their emotions. Even when they may feel a surge of emotions arising, they do not act on them. When the mind is quiet and stable, a person is able to handle their experiences with logic and reason. Emotions remain under control. One does not allow temporary feelings to take hold and determine actions. Instead, they are able to clearly make decisions by differentiating between right and wrong. They have control over thoughts and respond by consciously weighing options. Only someone with such a firm intellect can remain even-minded as they interact with the world.

KEY VEDIC CONCEPTS: *Avarana, Buddhi, Shama, Vikshepa*

2.13 PURIFY THE MIND BY REMOVING LIKES AND DISLIKES.

Our behavior changes according to our perception of an object or situation. If we like something, we find the feeling pleasurable and want more of it. If we dislike something, we find the feeling painful and desire less of it. The mind keeps oscillating between craving enjoyment and avoiding displeasure. As a result, the mind never knows peace. When one stubbornly holds on to preferences, the mind feels agitated when it cannot have that object or experience. Equally, when one cannot remove irritation, restlessness overtakes the mind.

Unfortunately, even successfully being able to enjoy comforts and escape discomforts doesn't last long until the mind becomes occupied again with the same dilemma. Likes and dislikes keep changing with time and circumstance. What one feels inclined toward today may be something that they are trying to escape tomorrow.

One has to overcome the fluctuations of the mind to realize true freedom. Complete awareness can be experienced only when past impressions and expectations of outcome do not determine behavior.

The mind focuses on higher thinking and living when

it becomes free from attachment to pleasure and pain. One becomes fully attentive having overcome the turbulent demands of the mind. Reason and logic prevail over emotional imbalance. An individual learns to see Reality for what it is and not what is projected in the mind.

A daily meditation practice helps to strengthen the mind by making it stable and steady. Someone who remains even-minded in pleasant or unpleasant situations lives in this world without worry. By letting go of rigidity, such a person remains flexible in thought and adjusts to circumstances. The more easygoing a person, the less agitations they experience. One comes to accept whatever circumstances are unfolding before them without judgment. As a person transcends conditioned thinking, they begin to treat everyone equally, give more than take, live by a moral code, and recognize social responsibility. Having overcome preferences, one lives peacefully.

KEY VEDIC CONCEPTS: *Dwesha, Raga, Vairagya*

2.14 PURIFY THE MIND BY REMOVING EGO AND SELFISHNESS.

When you do not even own your body, how can anything outside of it belong to you? Isn't it so that you will leave your body at the end of your life? Can you take it with you when you depart this earth?

What we call our individual self is the ego. My desires, my wants, my likes, my dislikes, my preferences, my hopes, my dreams, it goes on and on. We spend our lives exhaustingly describing our personalities and idiosyncrasies.

Ego here does not mean an inflated sense of self, such as giving oneself heightened importance. Rather, it is our attachment to our identity as the body, mind, and intellect. Ego causes duality and separateness.

This individuality we proudly display keeps us small-minded, fearful, and selfish. These false notions of security make us protective of people, objects, and circumstances to the point of pettiness. Taking things personally, fighting over status and reputation, becoming angry when someone insults or defames us, all result from this I-feeling.

What differentiation exists between us when we originate from the same source? How can individuality exist when we are all divine consciousness? What is there to desire, be jealous of, or compete for?

Only when we realize our true nature to be that one with all of existence does our entanglement with the body, mind, and intellect end. When we experience for ourselves that supreme awareness, that one which resides in all of us at all times but covered by our ignorance, can we understand that nothing is ours. We give up the erroneous identification with the ego-self.

This body has been given on loan to us as a vehicle in which to learn our life lessons. Through the body we come to know our weaknesses and defects, so that we can work toward transcending them. We are not here to judge and change others, but to continuously engage in self-growth and personal evolution.

The body serves as a temporary container, similar to that of a jug of water. When immersed in a larger body of water, the water inside the jug merges with it. The water in the jug does not disappear, rather it becomes one with the mass of water. Similarly, our body is a vessel containing the supreme consciousness, but due to our focus on the individual self, we are unable to see this expanded awareness within us. When we shift our attention from going outward to coming inward through meditation, we experience the individual consciousness merging with the infinite consciousness. Higher knowledge goes from being something consumed on an abstract level to a lived experience.

Just like we need the mind to transcend the mind, we need to utilize the individual self to transcend the ego. Many people misinterpret renouncing the ego as forcefully giving up one's self-respect, confidence, and boundaries. One should not be repressing natural feelings that arise. Compassion should not come out of a spirit of anger, pity, or as a way to escape life or heal from trauma. This type of approach can have detrimental effects and lead one to regress. It goes against the very purpose of meditation. Rather, one is not giving anything up, but naturally growing into expanded awareness.

What you do during the day affects your meditation practice and vice versa. Engaging in selfish activity agitates the mind. Selfishness results from thinking that all my actions are toward fulfilling my own desires; that I am the only one who gets affected by my behavior, and I am the most important person. This false sense of authority and status excites the mind instead of making it calm. One needs to get out of the false thinking that what one does in this world does not affect others. Instead, allow the barriers of separation to disintegrate by cultivating deeper understanding of oneself. Our egos prevent us from realizing ourselves as authentic beings. It takes more effort to stop oneself from being kind and giving, than allowing the natural flow of inner light to shine through in our actions.

The universal love you feel for all should be arrived at through inner development and spiritual progress, not out of a compulsion to be an empathetic human being. The internal work and self-effort one puts into daily life should organically lead one to realize one's own omnipresence and omnipotence.

Selflessness is a pure expression of the heart. Selfless activity generates calmness and peacefulness within. Selflessness comes as a direct realization of oneness. In our world today, the idea of selflessness has been either misunderstood or corrupted. Selflessness starts in the mind. When we begin to think about what is better for the community, society, the country, and the world as a whole, we organically become selfless. We are no longer thinking about just ourselves and how we can get ahead of others. When we understand that we are not the body and our identities are not tied to name and status, it naturally leads one to experience Truth. We let go of pride and ego. We take into account how everyone will benefit, prosper, and become more peaceful.

Let others feel proud of their false attachments to

ego. What is it to you? It does not take away from your self-worth and value. Real happiness is not derived from arguing about how great one is or proving one's prestige. Engaging in arguments and fighting are considered to be lower functions of the mind. Rise above them by abandoning your individual identification and attachment to pride.

Real confidence comes in remaining in that higher nature as you are living your day-to-day life. Dwell in that supreme state of mind at all times. Such a person has nothing to hide or demonstrate, no pretentiousness of any kind. Use your energy to raise the spirits of humanity, not only in certain circumstances, when others are around to see it, or when it is convenient but by how you are living your life. Such a contribution to society far surpasses the meager attempts made at proving one's worth. This is what is truly meant by removing ego and selfishness. The mind should become so pure that not only do you recognize the divinity in yourself, but you see that same reflection in others.

KEY VEDIC CONCEPTS: *Ahankara, Asmita, Atma–Anatma–Viveka, Mada, Matsarya*

2.15 PURIFY THE MIND BY REDUCING AND EVENTUALLY, ELIMINATING DESIRES.

Let's say you are offered a piece of chocolate, but decide not to accept it. You abstain from eating it, not because you do not want it, rather because you feel it is bad for your health. However, the craving for the chocolate remains. Maybe later you find yourself still thinking about that piece of chocolate. You wonder how it wouldn't have hurt for you to have a small bite. Perhaps you hope that you will be asked again. You may even think about going out and purchasing it yourself. The chocolate is still on your mind. It continues to occupy your thoughts even after the moment of being offered it has passed.

Similarly, one can be sitting in the most serene and secluded environment for meditation, but thoughts of worldly desires can still occupy the mind. The mind feels agitated thinking about acquiring possessions and satisfying ambitions. Instead of directing thoughts inward, a person focuses their awareness outward in thinking about how it can please the senses. The mind cannot remain still focusing on new objects and different experiences. As a result, thoughts are scattered and one cannot concentrate.

Access to the higher mind is always available to us, we just do not recognize it due to our preoccupation with sense objects and material gratification. For this reason, we must work toward reducing, and eventually, eliminating desires. This means that if an object were brought in front of you there would not be the slightest thought that you want it. There would be no temptation, mental suffering, or inner battle for it. Your mood and attitude would not change. The mind would remain ever-present and balanced. However, giving up desires should not be forced upon oneself. Otherwise, cravings only get suppressed and keep arising, causing the mind to become disturbed.

Through daily meditation, as one gradually withdraws the senses from the external to the internal, a person directly comes to experience completeness within themselves. Fascination with the world lessens upon the realization of inner contentment. As a consequence, desires and expectations decrease with the understanding that the joy we are seeking outside already exists within. We demand less from the outside, making the mind available for introspection and self-discovery.

We often think living simply means depriving ourselves of enjoyment. However, a person can still benefit from the objects of the world by maintaining appropriate contact with them. This means not acquiring unnecessarily and overindulging in external pleasures. One can still experience material comforts, but not be overly attached and consumed by them. It is in directly realizing that the temporariness of the external world cannot bring any permanent joy that true inner freedom arrives.

Neither does doing away with desires mean that we should not be productive and contribute to society or have any type of goals. We are not meant to be inactive citizens of the world. We have to be engaging in some type of work in society. This is our nature as human beings. However, action should not be taken merely to occupy time or solely for pleasure. Neither should it be self-seeking. One should properly understand and practice right action.

Right action does not mean renouncing all actions, rather it means renouncing the attachment to the result of actions. This requires putting aside egoistic feelings while working on an activity. Even wanting to do good in society is a desire with expectations. Such a person does their work keeping the mind on how they will be affected. If the intended result does not in some way help others or improve society, they may fear losing their reputation in the community. Or, if they get the anticipated result, they may worry about not receiving credit for it. The quality of the work suffers due to attention being placed on the final result.

When the focus of an action changes from personal reward to the activity itself, a person experiences real peace. One performs with zeal and dynamism when they do not worry about the outcome of an action. Letting go of anxiety over the result means that whatever the effect, whether perceived as positive or negative, it does not disturb one's peace of mind. We put in our best efforts when dedicating any activity to our higher self or the divine, instead of thinking about how it will affect us. This shift in attention from oneself to a higher goal comes when desires are slowly reduced and eventually, eliminated.

The only way to permanently rid the mind of desires is to realize our true nature as not this limited body, mind, and intellect. When we no longer identify ourselves as the individual ego, everything attached to it, such as status and pride, lose significance. As long as one remains ignorant of the higher consciousness within, they will mistakenly continue seeking external means to make themselves permanently happy. It is when supreme knowledge dawns that incessant desires end. We cannot truly be at peace without eliminating our ongoing wants.

We all have desires. The best way to reduce and eventually eliminate them is to first accept that they exist. Only then can we honestly and thoughtfully assess whether they are helping us progress. It is better to face our wants head on than deny or suppress them, which can lead to suffering. Working toward fulfilling desires with the right attitude and positive mentality helps to exhaust them and ultimately, free the mind.

KEY VEDIC CONCEPTS: *Aparigraha, Avidya, Kama, Karma Yoga, Rajas, Spriha, Vairagya, Viveka*

2.16 PURIFY THE MIND BY DECREASING OUTSIDE STIMULATION.

Many of us keep our minds occupied to avoid looking within. We would rather do anything else than be alone with our thoughts. We find ways to distract ourselves to avoid examining the current condition of our mind.

What will naturally happen when for the first time in the day you are turning off the television, technology, music, or your own thoughts and attempting to meditate? When the mind has been engaged with other things the entire day, expecting it to be calm and quiet is unrealistic. It will be wavering and disengaged.

We are responsible for the ways in which we involve our senses. Unnecessarily interacting with the outside world increases mental stimulation and restlessness. Aimlessly entertaining the mind takes us away from realizing our true nature.

We even waste our energy on the number of thoughts we have, as they keep coming and we continue indulging them. By giving power to each thought that arises, our mind becomes agitated. Soon, we believe anything it tells us, whether is helps or hurts us. We become a slave to our racing mind. Whether we are using the senses in outside stimulation or whether we are engaging in wandering thoughts, in each instance the mind is not with itself. We have to decrease outside stimulation in order to increase energy for inner contemplation.

It is when we remove outer distractions that we can realize our innermost thoughts. No longer influenced by what is happening around us, the mind has a chance to know itself. What a perfect opportunity for contemplation, self-observation, and meditation. We open up the potential to discover exactly how we feel about certain situations, get to the source of our challenges, and realize our blockages.

In this sutra, a distraction is considered to be anything that takes us further away from realizing the divine self within. A person cannot begin to think about elevating the consciousness when the mind is externally focused. One has a very difficult time directing awareness inward when attention is being consumed by objects and experiences. There is no space for higher thoughts to enter when one is constantly looking outside of oneself for fulfillment.

We already have so many unavoidable distractions constantly pervading our lives. In eliminating distractions, we need to realistically consider what we have control over. We have to consciously think about those things that detract us from a higher state of mind, as well as those that improve the condition of the mind.

In your own life, you may have noticed how you feel more relaxed after closing your eyes and taking a few deep breaths in and out. Why is that? When you remove yourself from outside stimulation, attention shifts within. Bringing awareness to the breath makes us immediately feel calmer. The mind is not anticipating the future or dwelling in the past when it is concentrated on the breath. It is in the here and now. If one or two minutes can provide such peacefulness, think about what a daily practice can do over time.

We are quite capable of being completely present and giving our entire awareness to the majority of our daily lives. Not to mention, we can live in such high frequency and raised consciousness if we remove outside stimulation. When the mind is not distracted and is completely focused, we have the potential to create our most powerful and life-changing work.

KEY VEDIC CONCEPTS: *Dhyana, Ekagrata*

2.17 PURIFY THE MIND BY REDUCING THOUGHTS AND DEVELOPING ONE-POINTED FOCUS.

An unsettled mind cannot concentrate in meditation. This is why we spend time purifying the mind of worldly desires and attachments that cause dissipated thoughts. However, the mind doesn't become agitated solely because of negative emotions. Even positive thoughts occupy the mind. The mind can remain restless even when a person plans to do good in the world. There are still demands and expectations that occupy thoughts even if they are optimistic in nature.

Purity of mind does not equal purity of thoughts. Improving the quality of thoughts does not necessarily make the mind pure. The only way the mind can withdraw from the senses and become quiet is by decreasing thoughts. A mind that runs on its own and gives energy to each thought that arises has to be brought under control. We first need to reduce thoughts in order to gain restraint over them and then we can direct them to one-pointed focus.

The mind is akin to a lake. When waves arise from raindrops or pebbles thrown in, we cannot see the bottom of the lake. The water needs to be calm so we can have a clear view to the bottom. Similarly, the reduction of the waves of thoughts allows us to realize the higher consciousness, the one always operating within us, but that which we are unable to recognize due to our unruly mind.

Once the fluctuations of the mind become smaller, it becomes easier to develop concentration. Since we cannot immediately sit down and become thoughtless, we have to gradually keep letting go of thoughts until we arrive exclusively at one thought. In order for attention to stay in one place, we hold on to one thought, to avoid all other thoughts. For example, in the beginning of a mantra or prayer, Om is chanted to avoid all other sounds and thoughts. Then, the mind becomes quiet.

Single-pointed attention is the beginning of meditation. We not only have to withdraw the mind from the external, but we have to direct it to something higher. Merely withdrawing the mind will not make it stay in one place. We have to give it something auspicious and engrossing to latch on to.

Kirtans, bhajans, repetition of *mantras, trataka* are all ways of settling the mind. We need support in helping to turn the mind inward and give it one-pointed focus. Concentrating on a symbol, deity, or holding an image in the mind's eye give us different ways of internally concentrating.

The mind should be elevated by the quality of focus. The spirit should feel lifted. Does anyone have a negative association with the sun? Does anyone think of their own breath as contaminated? Does anyone feel low after chanting or singing about the divine? Images and symbols that innately represent positivity, light, and peace help the mind move beyond the boundaries of everyday thinking.

In the advanced stages of meditation, when one is transfixed in the higher nature, a person no longer needs anything outside of themselves to support the mind. Any object, words, or visualization used to guide the mind up until that point automatically disintegrates into oneness. When external means have served their purpose, the individual consciousness naturally dissolves into supreme awareness. One becomes merged with the infinite.

KEY VEDIC CONCEPTS: *Amatra Om, Bhajan, Dharana, Ekagrata, Ishvarapranidhana, Kirtan, Mantra, Niruddha, Pratyaya, Samadhi, Trataka*

2.18 PURIFYING THE MIND IS AN ONGOING AND CONTINUOUS PROCESS.

Purifying the mind can be considered preparation for self-realization. In this way, cultivating the mind for the direct experience of total absorption of oneness is a lifelong (to many lifetimes) process.

Purification of the mind not only happens in the beginning of creating a meditation practice or during a certain phase but also during the constant inner work we have to occupy ourselves with, relentlessly day in and day out.

While meditating, a person consistently works toward reducing thoughts, developing concentration, and quieting the mind. Carefully, the sense organs are brought under control. If the mind has not been properly cleared of impurities, it cannot be made firm, steady, and stable.

Meditation is similar to tugging on a rope to dock a boat. We have to keep bringing the mind to a point of concentration, to elevated thoughts, to noble goals and an ideal image. Steadily we move toward pure awareness. It is a conscious and continuous effort. A higher level of understanding can only develop when supreme knowledge becomes realized through self-efforts.

Meditation *should* transform one from within. Thinking has to change. The way you engage with the world has to be different. Attitude, personality, and mindset must all undergo a shift. For this to happen one has to be cautious of what goes into the mind. One remains sensitive and alert to regressing back to feelings of jealousy, lust, hatred, and greed, without warning. An individual continuously works to remove the source of desires and attachments. Gradually, a person lets go of false preconceptions of identity and ego.

Meditation is a practice that continues whether it is a weekday or weekend, day or night, raining or sunny, whether you are fed or hungry, calm or agitated, fulfilled or unfulfilled. Meditation happens every moment of every single day.

KEY VEDIC CONCEPTS: *Abhyasa, Nirodha*

2.19 THE MIND MUST BE PURIFIED TO REALIZE THE GOAL OF MEDITATION.

In meditation, we are guiding the mind from external attention to internal awareness. As we move from gross to subtle, we slowly develop the ability to let go of all thoughts to one thought exclusively. Even being able to observe one's own inhalation and exhalation requires transcending oscillating thoughts. Through this process, we begin to experience a steady flow of concentration. Gradually, we go from thinking of ourselves as a limited being to experiencing expanded consciousness. None of this can be realized without first refining the mind.

Simple suppression of lust, anger, greed, pride, and jealousy will not free the mind because these emotions will eventually rise again. The mind has to be reconditioned in order to overcome the fluctuating thoughts caused by attachment to our individual experiences. The mind has to be purified in order to become a receptacle for higher knowledge.

No matter how many times one looks in a mirror covered with a thick layer of dust, they will not see their reflection. Similarly, our true reflection cannot be seen when there are impurities in the mind. When the mind itself (the very tool we use to reflect our experiences) is contaminated, there can be no clarity in thinking and purity of consciousness. Completely wiping it clean is the only way to see the true, divine self within.

Purity of mind should be undertaken for the sole purpose of ridding the mind of impurities so that one may realize their true nature. No ulterior motives should exist. This is why in Vedic tradition, knowledge was protected in order to preserve its sacredness. It would not be shared with anyone who hadn't first purified their mind. If spiritual knowledge fell into the hands of those who had not done the inner work to receive it in the manner in which it was given, it had negative consequences. This is the state of the world today.

Many are using spiritual ideas and philosophies to further their status and power. This knowledge is being misused as a tool to gain wealth and inflate self-importance. In this confusion, many people are faulting the spiritual knowledge itself, but it is not the knowledge that should be doubted, rather the person imparting it.

True spiritual masters and gurus have refined their inner personality to the point that they do not accept money earned through corrupt means; they keep every commitment made, speak the truth, and perform actions selflessly for the good of humankind. One should not only be inspired by this potential for higher living, but should take these on as noble ideals to continuously strive toward. Only a pure mind can appreciate higher values such as forgiveness, tolerance, and patience.

A sign of spiritual progress is when one starts regaining the innocence of a child. This does not mean being naive and gullible, rather living with a pure heart. A person should live in this world with curiosity, vibrancy, and cheerfulness.

A heart without impurities requires a mind without impurities. The mind must be rid of negativity, judgment, anger, and lustful thinking. In its place, positivity, compassion, and loving thoughts should grow. When the mind is pure, speech is pure. Tender and kind words automatically flow from a person with a serene mind.

One should realize that they are on the journey toward the goal of expanded awareness and pure consciousness. We are continuously striving to live in an elevated and equanimous state of mind. This requires consistency and patience. Self-realization is completely within one's reach given ongoing self-efforts through a daily meditation practice.

KEY VEDIC CONCEPTS: *Dharana, Dhyana, Kama, Kaivalya, Krodha, Lobha, Mada, Matsarya, Moha, Prasanna, Shad-ripu*

2.20 WHEN THE MIND HAS BEEN PURIFIED, THE GOAL OF MEDITATION WILL BE REALIZED.

When the mind has been properly and thoroughly prepared by removing doubt, developing faith and one-pointed focus, maintaining a balanced and steady mind, regulating the senses, removing likes, dislikes, and ego, cultivating selflessness, decreasing outside stimulation and thoughts, and eliminating material desires, it will naturally slide into the seat of meditation and move toward self-realization.

KEY VEDIC CONCEPTS: *Atma-jnyana, Samadhi, Shat-sampatti*

CHAPTER 3

Developing a Practice
and
Overcoming Challenges
During Meditation

3.1 MAINTAIN AN INDIVIDUAL SILENT MEDITATION PRACTICE.

Daily meditation must be a solitary activity engaged in isolation. To dwell in the self requires exclusively spending time with the mind. There must exist the proper condition in which to give sole attention to the inner nature.

From ancient times, yogis have closed themselves off from the outer world in places like the mountains, woods, and caves. Removed from the distractions of everyday life, they were able to explore the confines of the mind and make incredible breakthroughs in understanding the highest nature of human beings.

If we logically think about the practical purpose an isolated place serves, we realize that it helps in creating the time for meditation without distractions from human contact or outside stimulation. We cannot purposefully spend time with ourselves while interacting with the world. Withdrawing the senses from external elements helps the mind to focus on itself and recognize the presence of awareness within.

A person does not have to take such extreme measures as to travel to far parts of the world and live in remote places to create a similar atmosphere. One can cultivate similar conditions within their current environment. This could mean meditating alone inside of a room for a few minutes or at a time when there is the least amount of outside noise. Solitude should be embraced willingly, not out of fear or compulsion. It should give an individual a renewed sense of self. A person should be able to sit quietly without feeling restless and agitated.

Although a person may choose to play music or listen to guided meditations, this should be done as preparation for silently sitting in meditation. One should give oneself the opportunity to sit quietly afterwards and merge with the serenity they are feeling.

Making time to be alone with the mind also helps us have a different level understanding of ourselves. This is something that we may not be familiar with or even realize exists. We are able to see ourselves outside of the everyday labels and boxes we inevitably judge our progress by, usually dictated by others and the culture we live in. We gain an expansive view of our life. This leads to clarity in thinking. The silence helps guide us in elevating our minds and setting higher goals.

This does not mean a person should not meditate in a group. Meditating with other people may help give someone the motivation and support to keep a regular practice. Especially, if surrounded by those who are more spiritually advanced, it can help raise a person's energy and provide direction to an aspirant.

However, in addition, one must also continue maintaining their own practice. A person's meditation routine should remain consistent and ongoing, no matter the outer involvements. One need not necessarily exclude other methods and tools, but should be mindful to keep up with the same individualized meditation technique they have been practicing.

Neither does having a personal practice mean that one should remain isolated. Once you have your time for meditation, quiet inner reflection, and contemplation, you should go out into the world. Our experiences are the testing ground for our meditations. Each series of life events helps us evolve by indicating to us what still needs to be worked on within ourselves. It is only by knowing our deficiencies that we can properly overcome them and move toward higher understanding.

KEY VEDIC CONCEPTS: *Sadhaka, Sadhana*

3.2 MAINTAIN THE SAME PLACE, TIME, AND DURATION FOR MEDITATION.

People travel around the world looking for an ideal environment in which to meditate. Some go in search of a holy place or attend retreats in far off destinations. Although there are certain environments that are spiritually charged and can temporarily motivate someone to meditate, an internal transformation can only take place through consistent self-efforts over a long period of time. It should not be that one makes great efforts while in a specific location, but then loses that same motivation when at home.

Every effort should be made to not alter your daily meditation practice due to time and space. One does not forego brushing their teeth or eating meals because of traveling or staying in a different place. Similarly, your meditation practice should not be stopped because you are not at home. One must have regularity to progress in meditation no matter where they are living. Nothing should divert you from keeping the same dedicated spiritual routine every day. This takes conviction, dedication, and strength of mind, which have to be developed and maintained over a period of time.

Ideally, a person who is serious about their meditation practice and spiritual growth should not leave a comfortable home environment to go to a place where they have to struggle to meet basic daily needs. If it is possible, one should remain in one place, turn their attention inwards, and diligently work toward creating a steady meditation practice. Moving from one place to another adds unnecessary distractions and dissipates energy that could otherwise be used for meditation. One has to adjust to a new environment and familiarize oneself with a different location. Practical and logistical matters consume vitality. The energy required to remove distractions and adjust to unanticipated situations can be better utilized in actually meditating.

Meditating at the same time every day helps make meditation a part of a daily habit. There are four optimal times for meditation: before or during sunrise, noon, sunset, and midnight. These represent the transitions in the day. As the sun goes through its phases, we also should be moving through the cycles of the day from morning spiritual practice, to afternoon activity in the world, to evening resting and spending time with family, to nightly inner reflection and quietude. Ancient yogis also found through their own meditations that sitting during these times made it less challenging to concentrate and quiet the mind due to the vibrational energy of the earth.

However, it must be said that being unable to meditate during one of these auspicious times should not deter someone from meditating at all. At first, an individual should find a suitable time to meditate that is convenient and fits into their lifestyle and schedule. Creating a consistent meditation practice is most important. Then, one can work toward meditating at a time of their choosing.

As one progresses, they will naturally come to realize that it is not enough to keep up with a daily practice, but they also need to maintain the duration of meditation developed up until that point. Substituting too many shorter meditations when limited on time interrupts focus and eventually disrupts the flow of a daily practice. For instance, when one has been organically able to grow a focused ten-minute daily meditation habit but due to time restrictions begins doing shorter meditations in order to not lose consistency, this will stagnate self-development.

Sometimes circumstances require adjusting one's meditation practice. However, varying a regular meditation routine frequently adversely affects progress. Every attempt should be made to not go backwards, but keep moving forward.

It is very important to maintain the same meditation routine on a daily basis. Any modifications made should be temporary. To quiet the mind, develop concentration, and transcend into higher consciousness requires applying the exact same methods every day. To naturally evolve into this elevated state requires a disciplined practice.

KEY VEDIC CONCEPTS: *Ananya-manas, Sadhana*

3.3 MAKE TIME FOR THINKING.

For most people, thoughts seem to increase while attempting to quiet the mind. In meditation, memories we had long forgotten about come up. Unsettled feelings we assumed to be resolved and properly dealt with rise to the surface. We remember experiences we had no idea made an impact on us. We recall moments we did not even realize were part of our subconscious.

Due to the mind not being given dedicated time to be with itself, thoughts that were suppressed by outside stimulation and distraction are all of a sudden given freedom to run wild during meditation. The undisciplined mind desires to know silence, but cannot because of its conditioning and habits. One way to tame these thoughts and prevent them from overpowering the mind while meditating is to make time for thinking outside of meditation.

Making time to think gives us a chance to digest all that has happened in the day. It helps us to become clear about our feelings. When we give the mind space to freely flow, without restrictions, it decreases the chances of the mind wandering during meditation. A person can choose whatever method they find pleasing to let out their thoughts, such as writing or going for a walk.

One should allow oneself time to organically think, without judgment or suppression. It does not matter if thoughts are considered positive or negative, happy or sad, angry or peaceful. All emotions should be embraced, so that they can be openly confronted and processed.

Carving out specific time for thinking about whatever is coming up in the mind decreases the chance of it arising in meditation. It becomes less challenging to be present and attentive, as well as develop focus, when one sits to meditate. Thinking should eventually turn into self-observation and reflection, not only about our individual selves, but our higher nature.

KEY VEDIC CONCEPTS: *Vichar*

3.4 MAKE TIME FOR REFLECTION AND SELF-INQUIRY.

A person cannot spiritually evolve without reflection and self-inquiry. Any movement forward requires introspection. A person has to see that there is a need for change in order to create change.

Why do you think the way you do? Why do you have certain habits? Why do you like some things and dislike other things? Why do you react the way you do in specific situations? Why do you have particular tendencies?

In meditation, as we are attempting to make the unconscious, conscious, we can help along our progress by also making time for self-analysis. This demands a more intentional and structured type of being with oneself than in meditation or during the time we make for thinking. We may do this by recalling, at the end of the day, each one of our activities so as to understand how we spent our time. This can further help us evaluate our habits and tendencies. We can practice journaling by answering specific questions that prompt us to understand ourselves in a deeper way. This can help us to visually see our patterns of thinking and our current emotional state. These are only a couple of ideas about how we can practically implement time for reflection into our lives.

Hidden memories, surprising emotions, unrealized desires, the uncertainty of what is stored in the mind prevents many individuals from even trying to find out. However, openly confronting our feelings through ongoing introspection ultimately helps us remove our inner barriers to realizing real happiness. This process cannot be avoided on the path to liberation.

We have to first accept ourselves completely. This includes acknowledging all of our perceived negative and positive thoughts. We must be open to accepting ourselves as a flawed human being who has the ability to improve through self-efforts. Then, we can move toward letting go of any limitations that are keeping us from realizing our higher self.

Daily meditation helps us to evaluate ourselves from a balanced mind. Through an everyday practice, we come to spontaneously observe ourselves while interacting with the world. An individual naturally begins to wonder if the words they are speaking are aligned with how they are feeling and thinking. One begins to automatically evaluate the intentions behind what they are saying. A person starts to notice the condition of their mind, whether it is agitated, overexcited, disturbed, calm, or quiet. One becomes a witness to their thoughts. When in the midst of the objects of the world, a person starts to become aware of the things they are getting attracted to and what types of desires are arising. An individual begins to notice the kinds of topics of conversations they are having with others and if it is helping to elevate the mind or cause further restlessness. One becomes more attentive of their actions and the types of activities they are engaging in.

We cannot force this type of self-analysis. However, we can begin by making time for introspection in the best way we know how alongside meditating every day. As we progress in our meditations, we will notice how the level of our mindset evolves. Our thinking becomes increasingly sharp and narrowly subtle. We ask ourselves more refined and deeper questions. It is through both keeping up with our daily meditation practice and making time for self-observation that we reach higher stages of self-development.

KEY VEDIC CONCEPTS: *Ahimsa, Sakshi, Vichar*

3.5 CONCENTRATION IS ONLY A STEP IN MEDITATION: NOT THE FINAL GOAL.

The mind will not be still and void of thoughts as soon as one begins to meditate. The consciousness has to be given a basis to dwell in as support in meditation. The mind can be helped along in developing concentration by bringing attention to either something outside of us, like an object or a natural element, or within us, such as a mantra or the breath. Any symbol, image, or words utilized in meditation helps to bring scattered thoughts into one sole focus.

At this stage, the mind is aware that it is attempting to bring thoughts to one line of thinking. Intentionally directing thoughts still keeps us confined to the limitations of the senses. One should not falsely believe they have reached the culmination of their meditation practice when they are able to steadily hold the mind in one place.

Words or the image we remain focused on during meditation eventually disintegrates into expanded awareness. Naturally, the unbroken flow of concentration leads to total absorption. As we get closer to realizing oneness, we feel like removing the body like a heavy coat we are wearing. One feels light and free when immersed in transcendence. The feeling of the physical form disappears. We feel neither male nor female. We merge with the infinite, no beginning, no end. The feeling of total bliss absorbs the self. No worldly feeling comes close to it. Nothing outside of ourselves could ever produce this kind of elation. With ego transcended, the final result of meditation is realized.

Concentration serves as a necessary phase and temporary means on the path to realizing ultimate peace. It gives us support in moving beyond human realms of knowing. By steadily reaching higher levels of meditation through one's own practice, our separate identity dissolves into oneness. One has to transcend the individual consciousness to experience self-realization. Therefore, concentration needs to be understood in its proper place in meditation.

KEY VEDIC CONCEPTS: *Anadi–ananta, Dharana, Dhyana, Ishta Devata, Ishvarapranidhana, Roopa*

3.6   ACCEPT SUPPORT.

Do not let pride get in the way of accepting support in your meditation practice. If tools are available for you to deepen and strengthen your daily practice, make use of them. Do not stubbornly overlook these items or guides. Do not let your self-importance get the best of your common sense in receiving help. Adopt methods that will make your meditation practice less challenging.

In the beginning of creating an everyday meditation practice, you may need several cushions to feel comfortable in your seated posture. You may need to listen to guided meditations to make you feel calmer. You may need to practice *yogasana* to prepare your body and mind. Chanting before meditation may help put you in a meditative mindset. Experiment and understand what suits your personality and temperament. What do you find the most helpful to your needs?

You must start small and accept help to create a sustainable meditation practice. Being able to meditate for a long period of time and transcending the confines of the mind does not happen easily. For most people, these are goals that are only reached after consistent self-efforts over a significant period of time. These are the realities of creating a practice. Accepting that daily meditation is a process that takes continuous work will help one move through the different stages of progress with patience.

As one advances in their practice, naturally they will become less dependent on external aids. There could even be a possibility that any outside stimulation starts feeling like a distraction. A person may find the smell of incense or the sound of music prevents them from developing concentration.

One thing should be stated: despite any number of outside tools used, time for silent meditation should always be kept. One can practice measured breathing, journaling, *Japa Mala* Meditation, but nothing compares to sitting quietly with the mind. Whatever is practiced with the support of objects helps to lessen thoughts and bring awareness to one point. This preparation for meditation is necessary, especially when one is new to creating and maintaining a practice.

However, real meditation means being silent with oneself without any external stimulation. One must be able to sit alone with the mind to dwell in the higher self. Change, growth, and evolution happen by realizing and working toward slowly uncovering the divine within oneself.

Beginner tools should not become a crutch. One should not become dependent on them to meditate.

However, neither should there be any shame in utilizing them or an expectation to do away with them as soon as possible. One needs support when developing any new habit or skill. A child has to hold the hand of a parent while crossing the street until it develops the maturity and understanding to be able to do it by themselves. This is a necessary part of life for cultivating independence in an individual.

Similarly, one needs guidance in meditation until one begins to experience the benefits and gains personal understanding. It is through this direct realization alone that one will no longer need external help. The time needed for this will be different for each individual.

As a person begins to get closer to their divine nature, they naturally feel motivated to sit every day. When one discovers serenity and peace within oneself, automatically the need for any outside support drops off.

KEY VEDIC CONCEPTS: *Japa Mala Meditation, Yogasana*

3.7 MAINTAIN HEALTH OF THE PHYSICAL BODY.

We have to continuously work on the body to prevent it from becoming an impediment to our progress in meditation. This is done by taking care of it. Without a healthy body, not only are we limited physically, but we also have little energy to cultivate the mind. If we are ill or in physical pain, the mind becomes focused on healing the body, not transcending to a higher state. Most of our energy goes into becoming vital again. We want to make sure that we have the energy to focus on inner spiritual development.

Keeping the body strong also helps us to maintain our meditation posture. When we are able to sit straight and upright, we remain more alert while meditating. The eyes have less of a chance of wavering. Where the eyes go, the mind goes. With the body steady, we are better able to keep the eyes either fixed on one spot or closed. This prevents us from getting distracted. It is important to have a firm and stable meditation posture in order to continue progressing. Ideally, a person should keep their head, neck, and trunk aligned while meditating. However, even one who cannot physically do so needs strength of body to meditate. They need to be healthy in order to guide their attention toward the self.

Yogic cleansing practices like *Jal Neti, Nauli,* and *Dhauti* are meant to clean out the toxins in the body to prepare it for higher practices. When we purify the physical body, we also purify our mental state. Additionally, the physical practice of yoga, known as *yogasana,* prevents the body from becoming an obstacle during meditation. One of the main reasons we practice asana is to prepare the body to sit comfortably in a meditation posture and make the mind still. This is why in the sequence of personal disciplines known as the eight-limbed path, or *Raja Yoga,* asana comes before meditation.

Not only must we maintain the health of the physical body, but we also must remember that the body is an external expression of the mind. If the mind is holding on to any negativity, or feeling troubled and agitated, the body will not remain still. Any meditation posture will feel uncomfortable due to inner restlessness. However, as we purify the mind, gain restraint over the senses, and reduce thoughts, we automatically begin to sit still for longer periods of time. Remaining in a constant flow of one-pointed focus, attention from the body transcends into expanded awareness.

KEY VEDIC CONCEPTS: *Asana, Dhauti, Jal Neti, Nauli, Raja Yoga, Saucha, Shatkriyas, Sthirata, Yogasana*

3.8 CONSERVE ENERGY AND DIRECT IT TOWARDS ELEVATING THE MIND.

We want to direct as much of our physical energy as we can toward elevating the mind. Otherwise, we waste the potential to harness and guide it toward spiritual endeavors. Some of the same energy we use in pursuit of sensual pleasures and material desires, can instead be channeled to meditate. This is not brand-new energy that we get from somewhere, rather it is utilization of the energy we already have, being used in a different way. We are merely redirecting the energy we would typically expend outside of ourselves and bringing it within.

Each day our physical energy gets spent in mundane activities that we normally do not think twice about. For example, talking uses up a large part of our vitality. A person who talks a lot has an active mind. Usually their energy goes into explaining their preferences, opinions, sharing stories, and describing experiences. They often have low memory retention because they do not listen when others speak, since they do most of the talking. They are unable to focus due to the preoccupation with their own thoughts. These individuals get exhausted by their inability to still the mind.

Someone who lives with inner tranquility and a balanced mind speaks very little. Their energy goes into being fully present. Having developed self-control, when they do speak their words are carefully selected. One may even observe that many spiritual teachers and gurus do not unnecessarily talk. They do not spend energy in discussing their identities and material problems because they have realized their true nature to not be this individual form. Always dwelling in that higher consciousness, their minds remain quiet.

Who we spend time with, what kind of work we do, how we spend the day, slowly uses up whatever limited energy we have each day. We need to mindfully think of how our energy gets used. It is important to honestly evaluate whether activities are helping us move toward or away from our higher self.

Additionally, what we choose to give our attention to each day determines how much energy we use up. One can feel either exhausted or relaxed by the quality of thoughts. Spending time replaying memories, fantasizing, and worrying about the future uses up vital energy. Whereas living in complete awareness allows a person to conserve their energy with the mind remaining in one place.

Even performing actions haphazardly, begrudgingly, or cynically, creates added effort. Keeping a negative attitude zaps one of spirit and dynamism. A scattered mind leaves one feeling fatigued. When we are tired, we barely have enough energy to take care of our basic needs. Where will we come up with the vigor and eagerness to work toward self-unfoldment?

When we keep the goal of realizing the higher self in our minds, then automatically all of our actions derive out of reaching that objective. The mind remaining in an elevated state of awareness greets the world with a positive attitude, cheerful disposition, and happy mindset. A person with evenness of mind does not allow their emotions to overpower them, leaving them with more than enough energy for completing their responsibilities and obligations. A peaceful person is not burdened by judgments and expectations, and is therefore able to give their full attention to each moment. It is only such a person that has the energy to dedicate to an ongoing meditation practice.

KEY VEDIC CONCEPTS: *Brahmacharya, Ojas, Vairagya*

3.9 EXPERIENCES LEAVE LASTING IMPRESSIONS IN THE SUBCONSCIOUS MIND.

Each time we choose *how* to engage the senses, a thought gets created in the subconscious mind. This is the place where memories are stored, reactions and impulses are based, and habits and patterns reside. Any images and words a person exposes themselves to goes into the subconscious mind. They sit on the surface of the mind, waiting to rise up under the right conditions. Many times this is when least expected. These impressions manifest as thoughts while meditating, either helping to quiet the mind or distracting it further.

When we meditate we are undoing whatever we have intentionally and unintentionally put into the subconscious mind. This includes the impure thoughts that have left a lasting impression, such as anger, greed, and jealousy. While we work on removing these impurities, the mind is further being fed present experiences that also become impressions that come up as thoughts during meditation.

As we engage with the world, we need to continuously be assessing what are the things taking me away and bringing me closer to realizing the divine self. The kind of environment we surround ourselves with, the work we do in society, the types of activities we engage in, all seep into our subconscious mind. Once there, it becomes very difficult to remove.

The subconscious has great power over us. The more we repeat a thought in the mind, the deeper an impression it forms and the stronger its will over us. Eventually, it starts to become a habit in the way we think and act. Without realizing it, this thought becomes our automatic default setting throughout life. We allow it to sit inside our mind for however long it wants without question, while it recedes into the deeper recesses of the mind undetected. For this reason, we have to change the mind from the place where these instinctive and reactionary thoughts dwell.

Daily meditation helps us to rehabilitate the mind by strengthening the intellect and thereby transcending the patterns of the subconscious mind. When the mind is firm and decisive, we make intentional decisions. By rewiring the brain to respond with more self-awareness, we slowly raise the consciousness and improve our actions.

Chances for us to get pulled down to the level of the subconscious mind are everywhere. We are surrounded day in and day out by ways for our minds to be consumed with anger, pride, and lust. It is easy to fall, but not as simple to rise. So, we have to constantly be working on keeping our minds elevated by directing our senses and activities in fruitful ways.

KEY VEDIC CONCEPTS: *Buddhi, Kama, Krodha, Lobha, Mada, Matsarya, Moha, Pratyahara, Shad-ripu, Vasanas*

3.10 REPLACE NEGATIVE THOUGHTS WITH POSITIVE THOUGHTS.

Someone whose mind is clouded with anger, greed, and pride has no space to think about something higher and virtuous. The mind remains too disturbed to be directed to auspicious thoughts. It is impossible to go directly from a negative mindset to realizing the expanded nature within. This is why thoughts have to first be made positive. It is only when the quality of the mind improves that thoughts can be reduced, and eventually, the mind made still to experience oneness.

Focus should be on increasing positive thoughts, instead of trying to suppress negative ones. When the mind is given something noble to grasp on to and move toward in meditation, gradually lower thoughts drop off. As we practice bringing our attention to our chosen ideal, thoughts become pure and elevated. Alongside meditation, we should also be supporting our practice by keeping our minds exalted through our senses and external activities. Slowly, a person progresses in eliminating negative thoughts.

When beginning any endeavor, it is important to start with a positive mindset because the path of that action will equal the state of mind from which it arose. This applies to our daily meditation practice as well. Each time we sit down for meditation, we should approach our practice with a cheerful, enthusiastic, and optimistic attitude. This upbeat and confident energy alone can take us a long way in maintaining a meditation practice.

The way we keep our own mind impacts those around us. It is said that the energy we give off, even while sitting at home and just thinking our daily thoughts, are just as, or even more, powerful as the actions we take. So, our mind has to be cultivated in such a way that our thoughts are positive, humble, egoless, compassionate, and loving, because it not only affects us individually, but also all of humanity.

KEY VEDIC CONCEPTS: *Ashuddha-manas, Krodha, Lobha, Mada*

3.11 MEDITATION NECESSITATES EXTERNAL CHANGES.

Experiencing higher realizations in meditation without taking any physical actions to reflect these changes can lead to very little progress. Daily meditation has to be helped along by implementing shifts in consciousness. For example, meditating every day while continuing to live in a cluttered environment, exposing oneself to violent images, and associating with ill-intentioned people, may provide a person with a respite from these areas of their life, but it will not rehabilitate the mind.

A consistent practice will make a person examine their habits, thinking, and behavior. One will begin to evaluate oneself through a more refined lens. These are all natural outcomes of meditating every day. There has to be an internal struggle in order for self-development to take place.

An individual should be prepared to receive and accept self-discoveries. This necessitates that one be flexible to change and willing to make adjustments. A person must remain open to modifying their outer circumstances to meet new levels of understanding. One should continuously be moving toward aligning themselves with their evolved nature.

An individual should not deny themselves the spiritual growth they are experiencing. Remaining static in conditioned patterns, recycled thinking, and subconscious actions keeps a person limited. Instead, through meditation we are attempting to get closer to discovering our expanded consciousness.

A daily meditation practice helps one to develop the courage and strength of mind needed to initiate new ways of living. This does not mean that one should suddenly renounce and abandon their existing life. Neither should this be read to mean that a person should become rigid and unyielding in their thoughts and behavior. Taking drastic measures without proper understanding can be just as harmful as living in ignorance of our true nature.

Rather, our association with objects, people, and circumstances naturally changes as we glide into elevated states of consciousness. In situations where the mind may have previously felt agitated, we now begin to feel calmer, and as a result improve our relationships. Where once we felt the desire to indulge in worldly objects, we may start to feel that we can do with less, and as a result reduce our consumption. We gradually evolve according to our internal understanding.

The real practice of integrating meditation into our lives begins when we align thoughts, words, and actions.

This means not only living in harmony within oneself, but practicing that same unity while engaging with the outside world. Examples of this include only saying what you mean, not going back on your word, and following through with what you say you are going to do. This is one of the most difficult things for human beings to practice in their daily lives. Only one who actively and regularly attempts living in alignment can understand how challenging it can be. However, it is by consistently trying that we come to understand our personal pitfalls and what more work needs to be done from within. One should never give up the pursuit to realize the pure self.

KEY VEDIC CONCEPTS: *Ahimsa, Purusartha, Viveka*

3.12 EXPECTATION AND ATTACHMENT TO RESULTS DETERS PROGRESS.

Meditation must be approached with a balanced and practical mind. Expecting a particular outcome or anticipating results deters progress. It not only takes away focus during meditation, but also creates frustration when certain effects are not experienced.

One should not get attached to any sensations and visions experienced during meditation. These should not be used as a measurement of progress. Nor should these experiences be misinterpreted as having transcended the ego or as having reached enlightenment.

Many times people think they have gained mystical powers after having experienced some physical symptoms and sensory reactions in meditation. Few go as far as to give themselves the self-proclaimed status of a guru because they falsely believe they have gained the insights to lead others on the spiritual path. This can be very dangerous to not only oneself, but also to others. Not everyone will have the same experiences, and even if people share similar types of occurrences, it cannot be interpreted in identical ways.

Even such true, rare spiritual persons in this world who have gained transcendental abilities and exalted prowess do not allow their faculties to distract them from reaching the goal of self-realization. Usually, others do not even know they have gained such strengths and powers. We should aspire to imbibe the same discipline, selflessness, and dedication of these individuals in our own spiritual journeys.

Not only does giving importance to otherworldly experiences obstruct and distract a meditation practice but so do expectations of seeing signs of progress. Although one will gradually observe inner changes with a daily meditation practice, it is the anticipation of it that should clearly be removed from the mind. Even when experienced it should not be given too much attention.

Expectations and attachments to results take one away from the purpose of meditation. Instead of gradually moving toward self-unfoldment and expanded awareness, it reinforces identification with the body. These create more cravings and desires. This goes against realizing our true nature as pure consciousness. In meditation, we are continuously striving to go beyond the confines of the mind.

The focus of a person of meditation should not be on what will be gained from a daily practice. Instead, one should slowly work toward making the mind quiet, gradually lessening thoughts, and patiently developing focus during meditation. That you are dedicating yourself to meditating every day, creating time to solely be with your mind, and contemplating on something higher; this is true progress. The feeling of calmness and peace will naturally be felt from within with such dedication.

KEY VEDIC CONCEPTS: *Siddhi, Viveka*

3.13 DESIRES CAUSED BY IDENTIFICATION WITH THE EGO-SELF WILL BE THE BIGGEST OBSTACLE DURING MEDITATION.

Ego results from the attachment we feel to our identity as the body and mind. This identification as an individual being makes us feel limited. As a consequence, the desire to feel complete keeps us searching for satisfaction through external means, only to discover that it creates more bondage and restriction

The passion to obtain material objects makes us feel restless. Wanting immediate gratification and sensual pleasures makes the mind uneasy. Even having ambitions to make a positive impact on society makes one feel anxious.

When attempting to quiet the mind during meditation, those cravings and urges rise to the surface. The mind continues to ruminate on all of the things it desires to accomplish and possess. A person may even feel as though fulfilling these aspirations are more important than meditating. One wants to hurry up and finish their meditation so they can get back to their involvements in the world. The mind begins to wander and daydream.

Thoughts slowly get carried away in regrets, memories, and worries. An individual begins to feel prideful and passionate.

As long as one thinks of this body as the be-all and end-all of their existence, the need to protect all that it has come to identify with will exist. Veiled by ignorance, one falsely believes their real nature to be confined to the thoughts and senses. Desires will naturally follow when one sees oneself only as a name and form. Pride becomes the driving force behind all actions. Having forgotten one's true nature of divine bliss and expanded consciousness, a person further indulges in temporary happiness expecting it to be permanently fulfilling.

This continuous yearning for worldly objects and pleasures creates the biggest hurdle to progressing in meditation. One may begin to get a taste of one-pointed focus and inner stillness, but as soon as the thought of the individual self arises, again the mind becomes dislodged.

These subtle and entrenched impressions manifesting as desires can only be properly lessened, and eventually exhausted, by realizing the pure self within. By regularly bringing the mind inward through continuous self-efforts, thoughts slowly decrease and concentration develops. Directing energy to noble thoughts and ideals over time makes the mind quiet. One begins to transcend their

association as a limited being and experiences that oneness with the eternal truth.

A mere suppression of desires cannot bring about
this internal understanding. In order to remove the veil
of ignorance that keeps us from realizing the higher
nature, the desires themselves need to be eliminated. Otherwise, they will keep coming in an endless cycle. The
same doubts, distractions, and challenges will continue to
repeat in a pattern of thoughts. The mind will continue to
feel disturbed and agitated.

However, since it is not always possible in everyone's
life to completely do away with desires due to different
obligations and duties, the various paths of yoga including *Karma Yoga, Jnana Yoga, Bhakti Yoga,* and *Raja Yoga*
have outlined techniques to bring one closer to realizing
their divine nature. Depending on an individual's personality, temperament, and lifestyle, each path provides
different applications and methods to purify the mind,
thereby helping one to bring awareness within and keep
it there.

When one abides in the higher self, all distractions
cease. While meditating, any thought of time or feeling of
the body disappears when we remain in that continuous
stream of oneness. Although we continue to live in the
body, we are no longer trapped by it. Having overcome

the conditionings of the mind, the ego dissolves into the eternal Truth, Consciousness, Bliss principle.

KEY VEDIC CONCEPTS: *Aparigraha, Avarana, Avidya, Bhakti Yoga, Jnyana Yoga, Kama, Karma Yoga, Mada, Moha, Raja Yoga, Sankalpa, Spriha, Svadharma, Vasanas, Vivarjit*

3.14 CHALLENGES CAN BE OVERCOME THROUGH SELF-DISCIPLINE.

The most common challenges in sustaining a meditation practice arise from laziness, time, hunger, sleepiness, obligations, and sexual desires.

A person becomes lazy about meditating when they are unable to see the benefits. Additionally, one loses enthusiasm when certain expectations go unrealized or results do not happen fast enough. Furthermore, if someone's meditation goal was to receive a solution to a problem or heal from a traumatic experience, once that objective is realized a person no longer has the drive to keep going. Lack of guidance and doubt also affect someone's eagerness to meditate.

To get over the laziness about meditating, one must consistently meditate. However, it is the patience and self-efforts required to stick with meditation that make it challenging for a person. Thereby, laziness continues.

This is why it is incredibly important to understand the purpose of meditation and the reason for creating a daily practice in the first place. To realize the eternal peace within we have to slowly work toward uncovering it. When we not only understand the intention but begin to have firsthand experience of it, we defeat laziness.

As a person begins to notice the inner changes, this encourages them to meditate more often and for longer periods of time. Someone who notices that they feel more aware, grounded, and optimistic will want to continue meditating. This in turn creates an even more dedicated practice. Observing these positive differences in oneself alone can motivate a person to keep going.

Having a regular and consistent meditation practice requires commitment. When a person feels they have no time to meditate, it often indicates that they need to honestly reflect on how mental and physical energy is being utilized. Time can also become a barrier when a person isn't living their life with value. Spending vitality on activities that further the agitations of the mind can be better spent on self-development.

If we consider our finite time and energy to be precious commodities, then we must value them like we value money in our society. We are immensely privileged to have the capacity for discrimination and the ability to choose how we apply our mind in this world. The way you decide to spend your time is either bringing you closer to peace of mind or taking you further away from realizing your highest self. One should assess how they are allocating both their time and energy each day.

Circumstances, financial considerations, roles and responsibilities, all factor into how we utilize our day-to-day lives. Obligations to family, friends, and the community will overwhelm a person and prevent them from meditating if a daily practice is not prioritized. Although our schedules may not always be under our complete control, managing time properly and appreciating the value of meditation will go a long way in sustaining a practice.

One also needs to satisfy sleep, hunger, and thirst. These basic requirements cannot be ignored, otherwise the body and mind will suffer. Hunger and sleep are not in themselves inherently problematic. These are natural needs that every human being has that cannot be denied in order to survive. However, knowing and accepting that fulfilling these basic needs can make maintaining a consistent meditation practice challenging, will help better mitigate their adverse effects. Sleep and hunger can become distractions if not properly managed.

It is impossible to meditate when one is feeling sleepy. Sometimes a person feels so drowsy that they wonder if they are actually meditating or falling asleep. Since meditation is a conscious activity, one cannot intentionally practice bringing awareness within when they are too sleepy to have any control over the senses.

In addition, one will naturally think of food when they are hungry. Thoughts will go to preparing a meal and wondering what kind of food should be eaten. Considering that a person should not meditate on a full stomach and ideally leave two to three hours for food to properly digest before meditating, this too will be a logistical factor in deciding when to meditate.

Sometimes needs can be taken care of immediately, so that they no longer disturb the mind while meditating, such as using the restroom or scratching an itch. Although these too should be avoided because we want to give our complete attention to our meditation, satisfying them can help us again quickly refocus the mind.

In meditation, we are attempting to free the mind with its preoccupation with the body. We cannot do that when all thoughts are going to appeasing bodily needs and urges. This includes thoughts of sexual pleasure. However, the more a person turns their mind toward higher thoughts and contemplates on the pure self, the more the body is seen in its real light. Composed of skin, bones, and muscles, this body is merely a vehicle to learn our lessons and help us move closer to our soul consciousness. As a person slowly frees themselves from the deeply imbedded impressions of the mind, the closer they get to their own divine nature and realize that sameness in everyone. In such a higher state of consciousness, everyone is seen as brothers and sisters. It is in realizing this oneness that passion, lust, and desire are slowly removed.

Daily meditation mandates self-discipline, time-management, and prioritization. A meditation habit will not happen without structure. We often think of self-discipline as rigid, authoritative, and forced. Some of us may even become overwhelmed by the thought of creating it in our lives. However, the reality is that spiritual progress only comes through self-discipline.

This is not any different than applying the same principles and skills in becoming materially successful. A person who wants to achieve any worldly accomplishment has to practice discipline in their lives by being organized and focused. Anyone who hopes to be prosperous has to be efficient and productive.

The ultimate self-discipline is having control over the mind. Responding instead of reacting, choosing to engage the senses in beneficial and uplifting activities, directing the mind to auspicious and positive thoughts cannot happen without restraint. Otherwise, continuous cravings, overindulgence, and unending desires take a person away from having any self-control. The senses lead the mind, instead of the mind directing the senses. Only when someone has learned to regulate their senses by strengthening their discriminative power through meditation can they intelligently interact with the world. It is this self-discipline that helps one to overcome the challenges in sustaining a daily meditation practice.

KEY VEDIC CONCEPTS: *Atma-anatma-viveka, Preyas, Purusartha, Shreyas*

3.15 DESIRE NATURALLY TURNS TO DEVOTION FOR THE HIGHER SELF.

A symptom of love is service. When we love someone, we are ready to do almost anything for that person. We engage in acts of affection and sacrifice to show how much we care. We are more than happy to cook a meal or move across the world to be together.

However, our relationships change with time and circumstance. Depending on the types of experiences we have, our feelings for someone can go through many phases and interpretations. The transience and impermanence of human life also makes certain relationships significant at different times. Even the trust we place in a guru or teacher has the possibility to transform from deep reverence to disdain depending on both our faith and the situation.

When every person has flaws and defects, including ourselves, we cannot expect to find sustained happiness in any human being. Disappointment, sadness, and grief will inevitably arise when we expect perfection in imperfection. The unconditional love and oneness we are seeking, whether we realize it or not, does not reside in another individual. When our feelings for someone can fluctuate and vary over time, how can any person make us eternally peaceful?

Yet, there is an immutable, all-powerful ideal that never gets destroyed with time and space. When we begin to develop the same kind of love toward it that we feel for an object of our desire, we experience an exalted level of intimacy and admiration.

To realize it, we first have to settle our thoughts and cultivate one-pointed focus. Visualizing a deity or a natural element, observing the flow of the breath, or silently chanting a mantra all help to concentrate the mind.

When a person starts to experience peace in their own quietude, desires for external pleasures and material objects gradually fade away. Slowly, eagerness to know the highest truth and ultimate knowledge comes like a dying thirst. The mind becomes absorbed in a stream of equanimity. Devotion to continue discovering this inner expanded consciousness takes root. The ordinary, conditioned love we know evolves to one of surrender in the absolute.

The philosophy and practice of Bhakti Yoga guides those who are more emotional by nature. Instead of suppressing or denying one's feelings, Bhakti Yoga helps a person direct their energy toward a higher ideal. When the heart and mind get lodged in the thought of the divine, the ego-self begins to dissolve. This refinement of the individual consciousness permanently removes anger, greed, jealousy, passion, and lust over time. Fear and worry dissipate through the realization that the external divinity one has been searching for has been within all along.

Only when we can see the divine in ourselves, can we see it in others. Recognizing that universal love already exists within oneself will naturally extend to all of humanity. That which is in me must also be in others. Without seeing this oneness and sameness in everyone and everything, true peace cannot be realized.

Love in its purest form not only means recognizing the divine in each other, but living it in the way we think, speak, and act. We harm ourselves when we reserve our compassion and understanding only for certain people. Instead, when we can transcend limited and confined ways of being with each other here on this earth, we feel more inner freedom.

This does not mean blindly showing affection to everyone without discrimination, dramatic displays of physical touch, or making people uncomfortable by going beyond the boundaries of what is socially acceptable. Rather, this means living with a full heart and being completely present in each moment.

This becomes possible as we purify the mind of conditions, expectations, and preconceived ideas. As the mind becomes more calm and steady, we are able to accept a person and circumstance for what it is. We live spiritually because we are spiritual.

The mind has to be slowly guided to dwell in the higher self. There must exist an inner longing for self-growth and spiritual expansion. One must believe that they can be better tomorrow than they are today. One must remove all doubts that real happiness resides inside of oneself and cannot be taken away by anything external. One must wholeheartedly be convinced that a more noble and auspicious self waits to be uncovered. By bringing awareness within, one slowly develops the necessary love for the self that is required to meditate every day.

KEY VEDIC CONCEPTS: *Bhakti Yoga, Shat-sampatti, Vijnyana, Vivarjit*

3.16 DO NOT SHARE THE EXPERIENCES OF YOUR MEDITATION PRACTICE.

It is natural for us to want to compare the results of our meditation practice to the progress of others. It seems to serve as a type of measuring tool for our own realizations and milestones. Especially when one has no other support or guidance in meditation, it is easy to look upon the changes others are experiencing as an indication of being on the right path.

But what inherently happens is that a person may think that because they are not experiencing the same results or seeing similar benefits as someone else, they are doing something wrong. One may wonder why they have not advanced as much as another person. Someone may begin to doubt their own practice. An individual may even dismiss their own inner work and self-development because they become focused on what others are seemingly gaining. A person may even become completely discouraged and stop meditating altogether.

You do not want to be influenced by others reactions and in turn, others should not be influenced by your results and experiences in meditation. As you continue your daily meditation practice, your realizations should not be shared with anyone else, other than a trusted teacher or guru. And, even this should be with the intention of asking questions and receiving clarification about experiences and misunderstandings. Your progress should be determined by reflection, inner contemplation, and self-study, rather than outside references.

Everyone has their own journey to the higher self. What will happen on this path cannot be predicted or outlined. Our bodies are finely selected vessels for our souls to work through our karma and finally reach ultimate freedom. Every single person's lessons will be different. This life is merely an opportunity to exhaust that which keeps bringing us back to this human form. To compare our spiritual paths with others is futile. Instead, focus should always be on keeping one's own mind pure, controlled, and elevated.

KEY VEDIC CONCEPTS: *Bhava, Karma*

3.17 YOU WILL REGRESS, BUT EACH TIME THE EFFECT WILL LESSEN.

Just when you think you have made significant progress in your self-development, something happens that makes you feel as though you are back to where you started. An unexpected situation or an offhand comment by someone makes you revert to conditioned patterns and subconscious thinking. Those impure thoughts you believe you had left behind, return. You find yourself repeating old habits and behaviors you thought were now a part of your past.

Uncovering the layers within ourselves toward sustained equanimity requires continuous, intentional attempts. You are constantly working on improving the condition of your mind. There will be progress, but also backslides. However, there can be no advancement without internal struggle.

With a daily meditation practice, even if you regress, you start to become aware of it. You begin to reflect and self-correct through small improvements. You take steps toward bettering yourself. In the challenges, you will notice how your mind has developed, how you come to see yourself differently, and what is required of you to continually progress. The very process of it changes you. It is in this journey where the real transformation takes place.

Redefining and restructuring our daily life to meet the higher realizations we are having about ourselves takes ongoing efforts. We slowly move toward higher thinking and living. We have to patiently work within the framework of our personality, circumstances, and abilities. Everyone will start from a different place, but the idea is to begin and keep moving forward.

KEY VEDIC CONCEPTS: *Abhyasa, Prayatna*

CHAPTER 4

Changes and Realizations
Evolving from a
Daily Meditation Practice

4.1 YOUR MEDITATION PRACTICE NATURALLY EVOLVES.

A meditation technique serves as a basis for the consciousness. It is a method to concentrate the mind and slowly guide it to single-pointed focus. The meditation technique we employ acts as a support for our mind, similar to training wheels on a bike. The technique one utilizes in meditation serves as a temporary tool that naturally gets discarded once the mind becomes still. We only need support in meditation insofar as it leads us to oneness.

If a person has chosen the appropriate meditation method for themselves, then it should be continued without interruption. One should consistently practice the same style of meditation until it naturally dissolves into quietude. Upon having integrated the personality into expanded awareness, a person evolves into an enlightened being. With the individual consciousness merged with the supreme consciousness, a person walks this earth with unbreakable peace, bliss, and compassion.

Nothing can discourage a person with this goal in mind from keeping a daily meditation practice. This aspiration alone not only motivates one to sit every day but also helps them quickly progress. An individual should continue meditating with the intention that the higher self will soon be realized. One who believes that they will reach that supreme state of divine consciousness, eventually will, no matter how long it takes.

KEY VEDIC CONCEPTS: *Sat-Chit-Ananda*

4.2 SELF-DEVELOPMENT GRADUALLY HAPPENS.

Sometimes one may place certain expectations and pressures on oneself to conform to preconceived ideas of how a person of meditation acts. For some reason, living in isolation, giving up the world, being happy all the time, never becoming frustrated or standing up for oneself are considered milestones of spiritual progress. This type of generalized thinking can be damaging and lead to harmful behaviors.

A person can come to feel like they are depriving themselves if they have not prepared the mind for self-knowledge. Extremism happens when one has not arrived at spiritual understanding through one's own self-efforts. Imposing viewpoints on others transpires as a result of identification with our ego-selves. Frustration and disappointment occur when we see ourselves as separate from one another.

A daily meditation practice brings about gradual self-development in a person. Changes in thinking and lifestyle are a natural outgrowth of meditation. A shift in attitude and mindset comes about organically, from having slowly done the inner work. Happiness reflects in the way one carries oneself, the quality of thoughts one has, and in the type of words spoken. A smile naturally appears on a person's face because of the serenity they feel, not only during meditation, but also while out in the world. A person becomes attractive to others by radiating a calm mind and glowing inner peace. Compassion manifests in spontaneous action.

Anyone who lives in equanimity cannot hide it. One does not have to intentionally make modifications. The personality organically evolves. Transformation does not happen due to compulsion, rather as a result of a consistent and disciplined daily meditation practice.

KEY VEDIC CONCEPTS: *Bhavana, Shuddha, Sthirata*

4.3   SELF-AWARENESS GROWS.

Most people think that happiness is a direct result of an everyday meditation practice. However, it is actually self-awareness that leads us to inner peace.

Daily meditation makes us more aware of the nature of our mind. Spontaneously we start to assess our own thinking and behavior. We become self-observant. Each moment becomes an opportunity for reflection and self-modification. Naturally, we begin to ask ourselves questions such as: Is what I am doing right now helping me to become a better person? What is the intention behind my action at this very moment? Am I becoming a better version of myself or am I regressing into old patterns and habits? Am I making someone feel better or worse about themselves?

In order to evolve, we must accept who we are in this moment. Personal growth cannot happen without self-awareness. Through this process, we reach higher and higher plateaus of self-understanding.

Self-awareness means accepting every part of our personality, attitude, and temperament, while patiently and consistently working toward realizing the higher self. From self-awareness comes real change. This is why continuous contemplation and introspection have to be engaged in, alongside meditation. We need to move beyond the self-imposed limitations we usually set on ourselves due to our preoccupation with our identities as this individual ego. This bondage creates in us the inability to realize our own true nature.

To truly live in the moment we have to let go of past impressions and personal agendas. In any interaction with a person, if we are focused on how it will benefit us, we cannot clearly experience the moment. When we have preconceived ideas of how someone will behave, react, or what they will say, it takes us away from being completely present. We cannot be mindful to what is happening in front of us without examining our own intentions, expectations, and judgments. When we remove these restrictions, we allow ourselves to fully experience the world.

We are not on this earth to correct others behaviors or change peoples' characteristics and personalities. Neither are others here to fulfill our expectations or serve as instruments to meet our emotional needs. When you yourself cannot meet your own standards, how can you expect other people to? When your own mind is fickle and unpredictable, how can you rely on others to be consistent and unwavering?

When the mind is no longer burdened with chaotic

thoughts of the past or future, a person can be completely aware of the present moment. When there is no anxiety or worry, we are able to give our full attention. When we let go of the impatience to arrive at a particular goal or the expectation to meet certain standards, we are fully attentive in the here and now.

Bringing our full awareness to the moment brings joy and gratitude to each day. We even begin to enjoy mundane activities. With a daily meditation practice, naturally each moment becomes full of possibility for self-awareness.

KEY VEDIC CONCEPTS: *Dukha, Dwesha, Raga, Samatva, Sukha, Vikshepa, Vivarjit*

4.4 YOU REALIZE THE EFFECTS OF MEDITATION WHEN TESTED.

This world is our testing ground. How much we have or have not progressed as a result of our meditation practice becomes apparent while we are living our day-to-day lives. How we deal with unexpected circumstances and unpleasant situations become the measurement of our inner development. We are constantly undergoing these examinations.

The lessons we experience in life are opportunities to learn about our mind. Noticing if we are able to restrain our senses when met with external stimuli or observing if we can maintain balance of mind while engaging with others; these are the telltale signs of whether we are moving forward.

Our purpose in life is to understand our own inadequacies and defects and learn how to overcome them through self-efforts. We are here to engage in continual self-analysis and work toward our unfoldment. The focus should remain on ourselves, despite the outer circumstances.

When we realize that the world is helping us in our

spiritual growth, we no longer desire to run away from it in fear, confusion, or disappointment. When we can remain just as peaceful in the world as in meditation, then we know that our daily practice is working.

KEY VEDIC CONCEPTS: *Samatva, Samyama*

4.5 YOU BECOME A LIVING EXAMPLE.

One of our main goals in life should be to raise our own consciousness. Love, compassion, and selflessness are natural outgrowths of realizing our higher nature. We effect positive change in others through our own evolution. It is through our own personal growth that we become an example of human potential.

Through a daily meditation practice we begin to view our life as a social responsibility. We choose to see our existence as an opportunity to help others see the possibilities within themselves. By living in an elevated mind ourselves, we reflect to others parts of themselves that they may have not yet uncovered.

We consciously work on keeping our energy positive and uplifted. We mindfully work toward being the best version of ourselves. We continue directing the mind to a noble vision. Even in our constant attempts to live by the highest ideals, we become a model of what is possible. We realize that our mere presence can be inspirational and that we have the ability to spread peace just by the energy we carry.

When every one of us has the power to positively influence others, why would our words and actions be anything other than encouraging, supportive, and kind?

Our speech should bring about the inherently good qualities in a person. This should not arise out of a desire to be well-liked or in expectation that the same sentiment be reciprocated, rather from an understanding that we are all part of the same Superconsciousness.

As we progress in our meditations, we begin to understand that jealousy, greed, and competitiveness are diseases of the mind. A true spiritual person wishes for others to accomplish their material desires. The sooner others gain the wealth and status they desire, the quicker they will realize that real happiness cannot be found within these lofty goals. Then, will they turn their minds toward spiritual endeavors.

Keep raising your own vibration. Make it a point to live happily and peacefully in this world. Contribute to the evolvement of humanity. Work on removing selfishness and ego, so that not only will you yourself find deeper meaning in life, but you will also be of greater service to others. Give people something virtuous to aspire to in this life. Learn to see the positive and discard the negative. Leave people feeling hopeful and vibrant. Live at such an elevated frequency that others cannot help but notice you radiating like a thousand suns.

KEY VEDIC CONCEPTS: *Lokasangraha, Prasanna, Prashanta, Satya*

4.6 YOU TREAT EVERYONE EQUALLY.

When we realize that one consciousness resides in everyone, we no longer see differences. Our behavior does not vary whether someone is watching us or not. How we behave does not depend on the position or status of another person or whether we are in a place of advantage or disadvantage relative to someone else.

We regard a saint and a sinner, a king and a pauper, a friend and an enemy, all the same.

Whether someone is insulting or complimenting us, we remain unaffected. Whether someone is a stranger or family member to us, we have respect and compassion for all.

Remaining elevated, equipoised, and even-minded, we realize the oneness in all. We treat everyone equally.

KEY VEDIC CONCEPTS: *Ekata, Samatva, Sthir–mati, Titiksha*

4.7 FOCUS CHANGES FROM EXTERNAL SATISFACTION TO INNER SURRENDER.

Oftentimes people will ask God to help fulfill their desires. They pray for a new car, home, or even a spouse. We should not mistake this faith in the almighty as surrendering to the will of the divine or being on the path of virtue. Rather, we are merely replacing the onus from ourself to a higher source to make us happy through external means and circumstances. We continue to feel miserable when we feel our prayers have not been answered. Some even blame God and wonder why they are being put through such difficulties.

Believing that there is an all-powerful entity outside of us that will make all of our problems disappear reinforces the idea that we are not in control over our own minds and actions. We come to see ourselves as less than, lacking, and incomplete, rather than already full. We move further away from realizing the expanded awareness that already resides within us.

However, when we shift our attention to building spiritual strength, we begin to see that happiness has always been in our hands. We can still practice our faith in God or the universe. However, rather than praying that our unending desires and expectations get fulfilled, we can instead ask for guidance in realizing our higher nature. That while working toward, helps us lose cravings for outside objects.

We can consider God to be the one who gives us the fuel to direct our mind in whichever direction we choose. Ultimately, we decide whether we want to indulge in the senses or bring our awareness within. We choose whether we want to live with restless thoughts or overcome the negative patterns of the mind. We make decisions every day that either reinforce our suffering or help us move in the direction of true freedom.

By bringing focus inward, we come to realize our ability to change our consciousness. By cultivating the mind to accept the inevitable circumstances in our lives with level-headedness and balance, we come to slowly understand that we are in control over our thoughts. Our personal experience reveals to us that we determine the path of our lives by the quality of our mind.

A person cannot get close to God or the higher self without quieting the mind. It is impossible to realize our blissful nature without first stopping the incessant flow of thoughts. In order for this to happen, one has to transcend attachment to their identity as the body and mind.

Otherwise, the ego will continue directing a person externally for happiness. When someone's focus remains on gaining satisfaction through the fulfillment of continuous desires, they will invariably experience an internal battle of highs and lows. It is by overcoming mental agitations that one begins to know peace.

Without this gradual development, one cannot come to realize the changeless and omnipotent Reality that exists within every thing and every being. It is only through inner tranquility that a person can openly surrender to the divine as either a form or as the pure consciousness within. This realization has to be experienced by everyone on the journey toward liberation.

Surrendering does not mean passive acceptance and complacency. It does not excuse inactivity and laziness. Rather, surrendering means having an unbreakable faith in the flow of life. This includes being able to accept each moment openly, without restriction or judgment, letting go of the feeling of I, and understanding that our own actions have caused the effects manifested as our life experiences. It also means doing your duty in the best possible manner without getting attached to the fruits of your actions. This type of inner freedom can only be lived when we have cultivated absolute faith in the divine.

No one can take away your relationship with God

or your higher self. When such a bond gets created, our entire life becomes enlivened by the spirit of renunciation. Faith empowers us to work in this world selflessly. It is only with the realization of our supreme nature that we can perform our actions keeping our mind focused on an elevated purpose.

We should reach such a stage of devotion in our practice that looking at a photo of God should be like looking in the mirror. You should see your own divine self reflected in that image. This is the reason for the presence of God or a divine being in human form, so that we can aspire to these virtuous characteristics and righteous values in our own lives. An idol is a symbol representing the ideal.

When you pray, you will begin to wonder, who is it that I am speaking to? If I am already the divine, then who am I asking for blessings and salvation? Instead of asking for help from an outside source, your prayers evolve into more of a commitment to live from your highest nature.

Obtaining noble values, gaining patience, preparing our minds to handle whatever comes to us with equanimity, these are the intentions we should be setting for ourselves. When we focus on auspicious goals, we ourselves change to meet these aspirations. When the mind changes, our view of the world changes. Our attitude cannot help but also evolve from selfishness to selflessness.

We come to expect less from the world, and instead give more.

Gradually, the mind changes from expecting our own needs to be fulfilled to wanting to see all of humanity prosper. When all people are able to meet their basic needs, we as a society flourish. Positive characteristics have the space to develop in an individual because the mind and energy are not being occupied with how one will survive. With awareness remaining centered on self-unfoldment, instead of outward gain, we bring about transformation not only in ourselves but to all of society.

KEY VEDIC CONCEPTS: *Atma-jnyana, Bhakti Yoga, Lokasangraha, Sharan*

4.8 LIVING A HAPPY LIFE MEANS LIVING A MORAL LIFE.

Immorality weakens the mind and dissipates energy that could be used in spiritual pursuit. Lying, stealing, and cheating causes restlessness and an inability to focus. Such a person has little control over the senses and indiscriminately gives power to whatever arises in their mind. The inability to exhibit restraint over thoughts leads one to act impulsively and behave reactively, thereby causing more suffering to oneself. A turbulent mind creates a volatile and temperamental personality. How can such an afflicted mind be directed towards virtuous thoughts?

Practicing the right values in life lessens the activity of the mind. It makes the mind calmer. It is only an equanimous mind that can be directed to higher ideals and a noble purpose.

What guilt can arise in someone who speaks the truth? What remorse can there be in one who keeps peaceful thoughts? What regret can there be in a person who remains satisfied in the present moment? What anger can there be in an individual who lives in gratitude and contentment?

A principled person stands out in the world as

someone of integrity, honesty, and truthfulness. Such an individual understands the right thing to do, and does it for no other reason than because it is the right thing to do. Expectation of reward, recognition, and acknowledgment no longer become the primary motives. One acts for the sake of bettering the community, without self-interest. Such an individual of elevated consciousness spreads happiness and peace wherever they go. All of society becomes spiritually inspired and uplifted by their presence.

KEY VEDIC CONCEPTS: *Asteya, Satya, Shuddha, Tapas*

4.9 RECOGNIZE A GURU.

There was a time in history when lives centered around spirituality. During Vedic times, as early as 1500 BCE, kings were taught spiritual knowledge because they were given the responsibility of protecting morality in society. The emphasis on spiritual education was not to gain status and wealth for oneself, rather to uplift humanity through cultivation of noble values. Can we imagine such a world today?

When we find those rare people of purity in our modern world, we doubt their intentions and question their motives. This happens because most people themselves are not engaged in their own spiritual development.

To be able to recognize a guru requires that one first step onto the path of self-exploration and inner contemplation themselves. Similar to only a doctor being able to discern and evaluate the skills of another physician, you can only acknowledge a true spiritual teacher when you are working toward realizing your own higher consciousness.

Only your own experience in meditation will make you realize the commitment required to rehabilitate the mind. Through self-analysis and introspection you will understand how challenging it is to overcome desires, restlessness of the mind, and remove attachment to preferences and expectations. Through your own daily meditation practice, it will become clear what kinds of efforts are needed to reach expanded awareness and inner freedom. As you progress, you will see how much work it takes to gain restraint over the mind.

Our most profound knowledge comes from first-hand experience. However, since it is not humanly possible to experience everything in this world, we have to rely on others' direct knowledge. A guru is needed on this journey because a person of enlightenment has walked the same path and transcended inner obstacles to realize oneness. This person serves as a guide to answer our questions and clear our doubts. They are living examples of our potential. They give us the energy and motivation to aspire to higher living. Since we cannot always surround ourselves with the optimal meditative environment, it's important to have a guide on this journey who will help us stay on the right path.

Gurus have dedicated themselves to living a spiritual life. Through self-refinement they have renounced sensual pleasures and gained even-mindedness. They are revered for their ability to transcend ego-gratification and materialism. A person of true renunciation no longer suffers from the fluctuations of the mind.

Gurus have reached such advanced levels of consciousness that they have overcome speaking ill of others, harboring jealousy, holding on to anger, and selfish motives. Such a person lives in this world, but is not affected by it.

It is only through our own experience that we can acknowledge these auspicious characteristics and virtuous traits in another individual. It will not even come into the mind of someone who is not on this path to notice these qualities in another human being. Nor would a person who does not participate in ongoing self-development understand the hard work it takes to move toward a heightened state of mind.

Someone preoccupied with their own thoughts, habits, and patterns has a challenging time turning the mind inward. A person whose attention and energy are absorbed solely in material gains and worldly pursuits has no available space in the mind for higher thinking. When someone is unable to see their own higher nature, how can they identify it in someone else?

It is only when one is working toward spiritual goals that they can recognize a person of wisdom. Someone who regularly engages in purifying the mind understands what it means to apply spiritual principles with great discipline and initial sacrifice. The more consistent and deeper a meditation practice, the better one will be able to recognize the right characteristics in a real spiritual master.

In thinking of making someone our personal teacher or guru, we need to first observe their behavior, speak with them, and ask questions. Finding a true spiritual teacher who genuinely wants to help guide you in realizing your highest potential will always have their own practice. They will speak from experience, give you tools you can use from where you are now, will not make you feel uncomfortable, will understand your struggles, will not belittle your progress, and will only share knowledge which they directly know to be true.

A real spiritual guide will never seek attention and accolades. Their egos will not be bruised because they have transcended the individual consciousness. They will not ask that you help them spread the word about their teachings. If it resonates with you, if you feel it helps you, it will automatically become a part of you, and others will also naturally take notice.

A guru will allow room for you to come to your own understandings. They will never say you have to do something, rather they will work with you from where you are at the moment. It is not a part of them to cast judgment or offer their own solutions. Rather, they utilize their wisdom to creatively guide others to find deeper insight and truth within themselves. The reason for their presence on this earth is so we can learn from their experiences. A genuine spiritual teacher encompasses all of these characteristics.

Nothing can ever take the place of the internal realization of spirituality. To make ourselves available for a guru, we first have to take the time and effort to dwell in the self. Nothing can happen without our willingness and perseverance. This is not the type of job that can be outsourced. You have to do it yourself. It is through direct experience that we come to truly understand the path to enlightenment and recognize a person who has taken this journey.

KEY VEDIC CONCEPTS: *Guru, Prayatna, Sadhaka, Sadhana*

4.10 MIND BECOMES QUIET.

There is something within us that makes us aware that we are constantly evolving. As thoughts transform from happiness to sadness, do we not realize these different states of emotions as they are taking place? As we grow old, are we not aware that our body is no longer the same as when we were a child?

It is the unconditioned consciousness that serves as the basis on which we make these assessments. It is the supreme nature that never changes due to time or space. It is like the soil that remains the same no matter how many different varieties of plants are growing on it. The soil supports all the different types of growth occurring, but does not itself change.

Similarly, we have self-imposed our identification as an individual being on the pure consciousness. When we overcome the constant cravings for objects and experiences, thoughts slowly lessen and the mind becomes quiet. The individual-self that has long identified itself as the ego no longer falsely associates as emotions and thoughts. Having removed these conditioned layers, we come to experience clarity.

When the mind becomes free of our conditioned consciousness, it merges with the oneness that has always existed. A person realizes what has always been there, but has been unable to recognize due to past impressions and conditioning. This is what is meant by the colloquial term of "emptying the mind." We finally see ourselves unfiltered through a clear lens. Emptiness is actually fullness of expanded consciousness.

In the deeper states of meditation, name and form disappear. In the beginning of discovering this pure awareness, the temptation to fight this thoughtless state will exist. There will be resistance to stepping outside of our well-known comfort zone of ongoing thoughts. We may even try to force the mind to think.

As we continue consistently meditating, we learn to let go and surrender. No such things as fear and anxiety exist in the pure consciousness. How can they with the realization that we are already the infinite Reality?

As self-awareness of this individual body begins to return while gradually withdrawing from meditation, focus automatically goes to the inhalation and exhalation of the breath because there are no thoughts to come back to having made the mind blank. We naturally come to observe the breath. We become aware of the automatic flow of our breathing when the fluctuations of the mind have stopped. This is actually what we are moving toward realizing when utilizing the breath as a tool for concentrating the mind during meditation. The limitations that we set on ourselves are due to our attention, attraction, and attachment to this world. By allowing ourselves to easily get consumed by these three A's, we move further away from our real nature. When we bring the same energy within that we typically use toward indulging in our emotions, memories, and worries, we begin moving toward greater realization.

As we peel off the coverings, the light within us that has been shining all along reveals itself. Emerging like the first sunshine that falls on a new day, what begins as a flash of light slowly progresses into a wondrous glow. The self becomes illumined with divine bliss.

KEY VEDIC CONCEPTS: *Jnyana, Sat-Chit-Ananda, Shat-sampatti, Svadharma, Turiya*

4.11 REALIZATION OF THE REAL FROM THE UNREAL.

Through continuous self-inquiry, contemplation on higher knowledge, and dwelling in one's divine nature, a person slowly comes to know absolute Truth. One who has realized that they are already complete and nothing outside of them can make them whole, lives in this world undisturbed. With this direct understanding, they are able to easily distinguish between the real and the unreal.

Where most people seek happiness by continuously acquiring objects and holding on to them out of a fear of losing them, a person of expanded awareness knows only ongoing suffering. When the majority keeps working toward fulfilling and growing their desires, the person of enlightenment understands freedom in detachment. Where one allows oneself to get easily carried away with excitement and passion, a person who has realized their supreme nature lives with emotional equanimity. Where most become attracted to the temporary and sensual, a person of wisdom continuously seeks to get closer to the permanent and unchanging. Where most people feel bored in daily spiritual practice, the self-realized person knows endless joy. A person who can clearly see between that which will bring permanent happiness and that which will lead down an endless path of misery, will always choose the path to the pure self.

This is the Reality we are working toward realizing through our own personal experience in meditation. When this light will dawn cannot be planned or determined in life. Therefore, we have to continue our meditation practice regularly until this understanding unveils itself as a result of our consistency and perseverance. Each one of us has the potential to reach this place of enlightenment.

KEY VEDIC CONCEPTS: *Atma-anatma-viveka*

4.12 WHEN THE MATERIAL WORLD BECOMES UNFULFILLING, YOU HAVE BEGUN YOUR TRUE SPIRITUAL JOURNEY.

The more we engage with the outside world, the less happiness we find within it. When a person realizes that sustained joy cannot be found in anything external because it only leads to endless desires and wants, they begin to turn attention toward the self.

You may have noticed through your own experience that it is very difficult to keep thoughts on the divine self while engaging in external activities. When you are socializing with friends, do you remember your blissful nature? When shopping, do you think of your supreme consciousness? One is too immersed in enjoying themselves to think of God or the higher self while out in the world. All of our senses are preoccupied in these outside engagements.

It is through the direct experience of inner peace in meditation that makes a person realize that nothing outside of themselves compares to the happiness found within. One gradually withdraws from external stimulation and moves toward self-development. This is when the true spiritual journey begins.

Such an individual may live like any other person, performing their responsibilities and taking care of their basic needs. However, they remain uninfluenced by the changing world. Although this person may still participate in society, they maintain an elevated state of mind in all of their engagements. One may even continue to enjoy themselves in outside activities and sense pleasures. But, having realized real joy, one does not rely on deriving lasting happiness from these temporary objects and experiences. A person who no longer relies on the outside world for happiness remains even-minded and detached from expectations. Instead, their awareness remains in the higher consciousness throughout all of life's activities. Ultimately, this individual realizes the same joy and bliss realized in meditation in everyday life.

KEY VEDIC CONCEPTS: *Vairagya*

VEDIC DICTIONARY

Abhyanga: Ayurvedic treatment; massage. **SUTRA 1.10**

Abhyasa: repeated practice. **SUTRAS 1.1, 1.3, 2.11, 2.18, 3.17**

Ahankara: ego; the feeling of "I." **SUTRA 2.14**

Ahimsa: non-injury in thought, word, and deed; one of the Yamas in Raja Yoga. **SUTRAS 3.4, 3.11**

Ajnyana: ignorance. **SUTRA 1.8**

Amatra Om: silence following the chanting of Om merging in Pure Awareness. **SUTRA 2.17**

Anadi-ananta: without beginning and end; infinite. **SUTRAS 1.2, 3.5**

Ananya-manas: undivided attention of mind. **SUTRA 3.2**

Aparigraha: freedom from accumulating, greediness and hoarding; one of the Yamas in Raja Yoga. **SUTRAS 1.14, 2.4, 2.15, 3.13**

Asana: posture; can refer specifically to meditation posture; one of the steps in Raja Yoga. **SUTRA 3.7**

Ashuddha-manas: impure mind; lower mind with negative impressions. **SUTRA 3.10**

Asmita: the feeling of "I"-ness. **SUTRA 2.14**

Asteya: non-stealing; one of the Yamas in Raja Yoga. **SUTRA 4.8**

Atma-anatma-viveka: discrimination between the Self and not the Self. **SUTRAS 2.14, 3.14, 4.11**

Atma-jnyana: direct knowledge of the self. **SUTRAS 2.20, 4.7**

Avarana: veil of ignorance. **SUTRAS 1.8, 2.12, 3.13**

Avidya: ignorance of the Self. **SUTRAS 2.15, 3.13**

Bhajan: devotional songs to the Lord. **SUTRA 2.17**

Bhakti Yoga: path of devotion. **SUTRAS 2.10, 3.13, 3.15, 4.7**

Bhava: feeling; attitude; state of realization in the heart and mind. **SUTRA 3.16**

Bhavana: feeling or mental attitude. **SUTRA 4.2**

Brahmacharya: self-control of senses; chastity; self-discipline in excessive indulgence of sensual pleasures; one of the Yamas in Raja Yoga. **SUTRA 3.8**

Brahman: creator of the universe; that one infinite consciousness; ultimate Reality. **SUTRA 1.2**

Buddhi: intellect; reason; determinative faculty of the mind. **SUTRAS 1.9, 2.12, 3.9**

Chitta: mind; memory. **SUTRA 2.9**

Dama: to control the senses; one of the Shat-sampattis. **SUTRA 2.11**

Desha: place. **SUTRA 2.4**

Dharana: concentration; one of the steps in Raja Yoga. **SUTRAS 1.9, 2.17, 2.19, 3.5**

Dhauti: cleansing practice for the stomach in Hatha Yoga; one of the Shatkriyas. **SUTRA 3.7**

Dhyana: flow of concentration; meditation; one of the steps in Raja Yoga. **SUTRAS 1.9, 2.6, 2.16, 2.19, 3.5**

Dukha: misery, sorrow, grief. **SUTRA 4.3**

Dwesha: dislikes, repulsion. **SUTRAS 2.2, 2.13, 4.3**

Ekagrata: one pointed focus; concentration. **SUTRAS 2.16, 2.17**

Ekata: oneness, absoluteness. **SUTRA 4.6**

Guru: one who removes the darkness (veil of ignorance); spiritual guide or teacher. **SUTRA 4.9**

Indriyas: senses. **SUTRAS 2.7, 2.11**

Ishta Devata: chosen ideal. **SUTRAS 1.18, 3.5**

Ishvarapranidhana: devotion to your chosen ideal; one of the Niyamas in Raja Yoga. **SUTRAS 2.17, 3.5**

Jal Neti: cleansing of nasal passages in preparation for meditation. **SUTRA 3.7**

Japa Mala Meditation: repetition of a mantra with a beaded necklace. **SUTRA 3.6**

Jivanmukti: one who desires for liberation in this life. **SUTRA 1.4**

Jnyana: knowledge of the absolute; wisdom of the Reality or Brahman. **SUTRAS 1.11, 1.18, 4.10**

Jnyana Yoga: path of Knowledge and discrimination. **SUTRA 3.13**

Kaivalya: emancipation. **SUTRA 2.19**

Kama: desire; passion, lust; one of the Shad-ripus. **SUTRAS 2.8, 2.15, 2.19, 3.9, 3.13**

Karma: action; of three kinds, accumulated from past births, results and effects being worked out in present life, freshly accumulated in this life. **SUTRAS 1.3, 2.7, 3.16**

Karma Yoga: actions performed while keeping the mind on God or the higher self; selfless action without any attachment to the result. **SUTRAS 2.2, 2.15, 3.13**

Kirtan: singing the glory and increasing devotion to God through shared recitation. **SUTRA 2.17**

Krodha: anger; one of the Shad-ripus. **SUTRAS 2.8, 2.19, 3.9, 3.10**

Kshetra: holy place or field. **SUTRA 1.16**

Kshetrajnya: the individual or the Supreme soul. **SUTRA 1.16**

Lobha: greed; one of the Shad-ripus. **SUTRAS 2.8, 2.19, 3.9, 3.10**

Lokasangraha: uplift or solidarity of the world. **SUTRA 4.5, 4.7**

Mada: pride; one of the Shad-ripus. **SUTRAS 2.8, 2.14, 2.19, 3.9, 3.10, 3.13**

Mananam: constant thinking; reflection on scriptures; second step on the path to knowledge. **SUTRAS 1.11, 1.17**

Mantra: sacred syllables or words which through repetition leads one to higher states of consciousness. **SUTRA 2.17**

Matsarya: envy; one of the Shad-ripus. **SUTRAS 2.8, 2.14, 2.19, 3.9**

Mitaahara: moderate diet. **SUTRA 2.1**

Moha: delusion caused by wrong thinking; one of the Shad-ripus. **SUTRAS 2.8, 2.19, 3.9, 3.13**

Moksha: liberation from karma and the cycle of birth and death; goal of spiritual practice. **SUTRA 1.2**

Nauli: a cleansing technique practiced by churning of the abdominal muscles; one of the Shatkriyas. **SUTRA 3.7**

Nididhyasana: profound contemplation and deep meditation; third step on the path to knowledge. **SUTRAS 1.11, 1.17**

Nigraha: conscious control of desires. **SUTRAS 1.12, 2.3**

Nirodha: restraint. **SUTRA 2.18**

Niruddha: controlled senses and mind. **SUTRAS 1.12, 2.17**

Nitya: daily; permanent. **SUTRA 1.5**

Niyama: observance; internal and external purification; one of the steps in Raja Yoga. **SUTRA 2.3**

Niyamit: fixed; controlled; consistent. **SUTRA 2.6**

Ojas: spiritual energy developed through conscious preservation of vitality. **SUTRA 3.8**

Prasanna: one who is happy and has a positive outlook. **SUTRAS 1.15, 2.19, 4.5**

Prashanta: perfectly at peace. **SUTRA 1.9, 4.5**

Pratyahara: withdrawing the mind from worldly objects and pursuits; one of the steps in Raja Yoga. **SUTRA 3.9**

Pratyaya: mental effort. **SUTRAS 1.14, 2.17**

Prayatna: self-efforts; attempts. **SUTRAS 1.1, 1.3, 1.7, 1.14, 3.17, 4.9**

Preyas: path of the pleasant. **SUTRA 3.14**

Purusartha: self-efforts in the present to modify the effects from the past and create a new future. **SUTRAS 3.11, 3.14**

Raga: likes, attraction. **SUTRAS 2.2, 2.13, 4.3**

Raja Yoga: eight-limbed path towards self-realization. **SUTRAS 3.7, 3.13**

Rajas: principle of dynamism, produces activity or restlessness. **SUTRA 2.15**

Roopa: form. **SUTRAS 1.2, 3.5**

Sadhaka: spiritual aspirant. **SUTRAS 1.4, 1.18, 3.1, 4.9**

Sadhana: self-efforts in daily spiritual practice. **SUTRAS 1.1, 1.5, 1.14, 3.1, 3.2, 4.9**

Sakshi: witness to our thinking, senses and actions. **SUTRAS 1.9, 3.4**

Samadhi: the meditator and the meditated become one in total absorption; absolute oneness; final step in Raja Yoga. **SUTRAS 2.17, 2.20**

Samatva: equanimity in outlook under all conditions. **SUTRAS 2.8, 4.3, 4.4, 4.6**

Samyama: perfect restraint; repose. **SUTRAS 1.12, 2.8, 2.11, 4.4**

Sankalpa: thoughts, desires, imagination. **SUTRA 3.13**

Santosha: contentment; one of the Niyamas in Raja Yoga. **SUTRA 2.8**

Sat-Chit-Ananda: unchanged existence at all times-pure Consciousness-absolute bliss; term used to describe Brahman. **SUTRAS 4.1, 4.10**

Satsanga: company of spiritually elevated individuals. **SUTRA 2.7**

Satya: truthfulness in one's intellectual convictions and ideals; one of the Yamas in Raja Yoga. **SUTRAS 4.5, 4.8**

Saucha: internal and external purity; one of the Niyamas in Raja Yoga. **SUTRAS 2.4, 3.7**

Shad-ripu: six enemies of the mind, Kama, Krodha, Lobha, Moha, Mada, and Matsarya. **SUTRAS 2.8, 2.19, 3.9**

Shama: control or discipline of the mind; one of the Shat-sampattis. **SUTRAS 2.11, 2.12**

Shanti: peace. **SUTRAS 1.7, 1.10, 1.14, 1.15, 2.8**

Sharan: total surrender; refuge. **SUTRA 4.7**

Shatkriyas: six cleansing techniques to purify and
prepare the body for spiritual practice, Basti, Dhauti,
Nauli, Neti, Kapalabhati, and Trataka. **SUTRA 3.7**

Shat-sampatti: six-fold virtues, Dama, Samadhana,
Shama, Shraddha, Titiksha, and Uparati. **SUTRAS
2.20, 3.15, 4.10**

Shavasana: corpse pose. **SUTRA 1.10**

Shraddha: faith; one of the Shat-sampattis.
SUTRAS 1.6, 2.10

Shravanam: listening to the scriptures; first step on the
path to knowledge. **SUTRAS 1.11, 1.17**

Shreyas: path of the good. **SUTRA 3.14**

Shuddha: pure; clear; untainted. **SUTRAS 2.5, 2.9,
4.2, 4.8**

Siddhi: psychic power. **SUTRA 3.12**

Spriha: desires. **SUTRAS 2.15, 3.13**

Sthirata: steadiness, firmness either of mind through
concentration or body through asanas. **SUTRAS 1.13,
3.7, 4.2**

Sthir-mati: a firmly established mind that does not
waver at all. **SUTRAS 1.13, 4.6**

Sthitaprajna: one who is firmly established in
Superconsciousness. **SUTRA 1.13**

Sthiti: condition of being steadfast. **SUTRA 1.1**

Sukha: exalted happiness, joy. **SUTRA 4.3**

Svadharma: one's real nature or duty. **SUTRAS 1.2,**
3.13, 4.10

Svadhyaya: study of the scriptures and study of oneself;
one of the Niyamas in Raja Yoga. **SUTRA 1.17**

Svapnavabodhasya: regulated sleep and wakefulness.
SUTRA 2.1

Tapas: austerity or spiritual discipline; one of the
Niyamas in Raja Yoga. **SUTRA 4.8**

Titiksha: bearing pairs of opposites with equanimity,
i.e. pleasure and pain, respectful and disrespectful
treatment; one of the Shat-sampattis. **SUTRA 4.6**

Trataka: steady gazing meditation; pupil cleansing
practice, one of the Shatkriyas. **SUTRA 2.17**

Turiya: unconditioned Consciousness (fourth state).
SUTRA 4.10

Vairagya: intelligent renunciation; dispassion. **SUTRAS**
2.2, 2.11, 2.13, 2.15, 3.8, 4.12

Vasanas: inherent tendencies; impressions of the mind
that cause desires. **SUTRAS 2.9, 3.9, 3.13**

Vichar: inquiry into the nature of Truth. **SUTRAS 3.3, 3.4**

Vijnyana: knowledge of the self. **SUTRAS 1.11, 3.15**

Vikalpa: imagination. **SUTRA 2.9**

Vikshepa: oscillation of the mind. **SUTRAS 2.12, 4.3**

Vivarjit: one who has given up desires and anger, in essence ego. **SUTRAS 3.13, 3.15, 4.3**

Viveka: discrimination between the real and unreal, changeless and changing, eternal and ephemeral, impermanent and permanent. **SUTRAS 2.2, 2.11, 2.15, 3.11, 3.12**

Yoga: merging of the individual consciousness with the universal consciousness. **SUTRA 1.2**

Yoganidra: light Yogic sleep with slight awareness, that state between sleep and wakefulness. **SUTRA 1.10**

Yogasana: the physical practice of yoga with different postures. **SUTRAS 3.6, 3.7**

Yuktahara: regulated eating. **SUTRA 2.1**

VEDIC DICTIONARY SOURCES

Bhagavad Gita

Self-Unfoldment by Swami Chinmayananda

Vedanta Treatise: The Eternities by A. Parthasarathy

Vedanta: Voice of Freedom by Swami Vivekananda

Yoga Vedanta Dictionary by Swami Sivananda